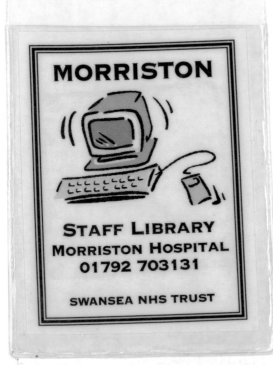

TOTAL REVISION FOR THE FRCA

2nd Edition

TOTAL REVISION FOR THE FRCA

2nd Edition

James Holding FRCA
Consultant in Anaesthetics,
Luton and Dunstable Hospital

Sarah Chieveley-Williams MRCP FRCA
Consultant and Senior Lecturer in Anaesthesia,
University College Hospital, London

Timothy Isitt MRCP FRCA
Consultant in Anaesthesia,
Luton and Dunstable Hospital

PasTest
Dedicated to your success

Egerton Court
Parkgate Estate
Knutsford
Cheshire
WA16 8DX
Telephone: 01565 752000

First published 2007

ISBN: 1 904627 93 5
ISBN: 978 1 904627 937

A catalogue record for this book is available from the British Library.

Text prepared by Saxon Graphics Ltd, Derby
Printed and bound in Athenaeum Press, Gateshead

Contents

Foreword

My advice to trainees preparing for the final fellowships examinations over many years has always been the same. First allow plenty of time to prepare in an organised fashion (about 5 months). Second look at the syllabus and make sure you have covered all of it. Third practise all aspects of the exam: the SAQs, the MCQs and the vivas.

This excellent book has been written by two of my colleagues (one a Nuffield prize winner) to help candidates with the third aspect of preparation. I was constantly surprised during my years as a fellowship examiner to find really quite knowledgeable candidates who had clearly never practised. They would run out of time in the SAQ or answer too few questions in the MCQ, thereby condemning themselves to fail by bad technique. Clearly they had not read this book which is an entirely updated version of the first edition published in 1998 (containing a completely new exam).

I once went to do a preoperative assessment (for someone else) on a distinguished professor of pharmacology. For want of something better to say, as I would not be the one giving the anaesthetic, I wished him good luck. "Luck has nothing to do with it" he replied. "It will be the skill and preparedness of the surgeon and the anaesthetist which is important." It is the same with the final fellowship.

Wynne Aveling
Consultant Anaesthetist
University College London Hospitals

We are always grateful for notification of any mistakes or discrepancies that appear in our books. If you do find an item which you suspect may be incorrect please notify the Publisher in writing so that we can ensure that any mistake is rectified when the book is reprinted.

Introduction

The new Final Examination for the Diploma of Fellow of the Royal College of Anaesthetists was introduced in November 1996. Details of the entry requirements for the examination, past SAQ papers and current exam information can be found on the web site www.rcoa.ac.uk or from **The Royal College of Anaesthetists, Churchill House, 35, Red Lion Square, London WC1R 4SR.** A Guide to the FRCA Examination: The Final, published by the Royal College of Anaesthetists is also available.

To be eligible to take the examination, a candidate must

- be registered with the General Medical Council
- be working in a recognised Specialist Registrar training post
- have completed at least 30 months' training in anaesthetics.

The Final Examination consists of a written Short Answer paper, an MCQ paper and two Vivas. All four parts of the examination are close-marked.

The scoring scheme for each paper is as follows:

1 Outright fail
1+ Borderline fail
2 Pass
2+ Outstanding pass

In order to pass the written papers and progress to the vivas, a candidate must score at least 2 for one of the written papers and at least 1+ for the other written paper. A score of 1 or below in any section of the examination will automatically mean a fail overall, no matter how high the scores in other parts of the examination.

The Short Answer Paper
This normally takes place during the morning of the examination; the MCQ paper takes place in the afternoon. Three hours are allowed for the candidate to complete this paper. All twelve questions are compulsory and are of equal value. Candidates who do not answer every question will fail the exam, so time management is essential. The examiners report that at every sitting many candidates fail to read the questions properly, and therefore waste time writing answers which can gain them no marks.

The College consider that this part of the examination is assessing 'higher thinking' and not just the ability to memorise facts. It can be difficult to show higher thinking in the 15 minutes allocated to answer, and so we recommend doing some timed practice answering previously unseen questions. This helps candidates to get into the rhythm of writing short answers, and forces them to develop ways of structuring and classifying the knowledge they already have. Answering four questions in an hour is ideal, most people can not concentrate for longer than that without the adrenaline of being in the real exam room.

In May 2006 the pass mark was 63%.

The questions tend to be classifiable into the following groups:

1. Paediatric
2. Pharmacology
3. Obstetric
4. Cardiothoracic
5. Guidelines
6. Pain (acute and chronic)
7. Intensive Care (theory / science)
8. Intensive Care (practicalities)
9. Clinical Measurement
10. Anatomy, as relevant to regional blocks
11. Anaesthesia for big operations
12. Anaesthesia for special patient groups (e.g. trauma)
13. Pre-operative assessment and investigations

Where possible the SAQs are broken down into sections and the approximate percentage of marks allocated to each section is shown. A strict marking system applies for key points within each question which is marked out of 20 with 2 marks for general impression and coherence.

The MCQ Paper
Three hours are allowed for the candidate to complete 90 multiple choice questions.

It is common for candidates to come away from this part of the exam saying things like "that was odd", or "even if I had all my books in there I would have only been able to answer half the questions". Some of the reason for this is that the MCQs are used by the College to assess breadth of knowledge, and instead of drawing new questions from the same old topics and textbooks the examiners look to the darker corners of the syllabus.

The College set very sophisticated exams, which show that they understand the theory behind good multiple choice questions. A perfect MCQ stem comes with a couple of statements which are quite easy (although the wording may be twisted to try and confuse or trick), and couple of statements which are hard (which only the better candidate will be able to answer) and one part which is almost impossible. Of course as the candidate it is not always easy to see which ones the easy questions are. The number of correct statements will also be random (between 0 and 5), but will tend to even out to half across the whole paper. Computer analysis of all the marks highlights any parts where candidates scored unexpectedly poorly (usually because the wording was ambiguous) and these parts are removed before the final totals are calculated. The pass mark, with negative marking, is usually around 55%.

When revising with MCQ books remember that the aim is to get about 60%, and try not to get bogged down in the minute details of the very hardest part of a question. Most people make 5-10 mistakes per MCQ paper on easy questions they knew the answer to because they did not read the question closely enough or simply ticked the wrong box. So there is an extra 5% there for candidates who can get used to concentrating hard and avoid slips.

In revising the MCQs for this book we have taken the syllabus as the starting point to try and replicate the feel of the real Final FRCA MCQ. Each paper has approximately the following balance of topics:

- 10 questions on clinical measurement/physics
- 20 questions on medicine and surgery
- 20 questions on intensive care
- 40 questions on pain and anaesthesia

The Vivas

If you achieve an adequate score in the two written papers you will be invited to attend the vivas. These take place at the Royal College four to five weeks after the written examination. In any given viva session all candidates are asked the same questions.

Viva 1 - The Clinical Viva (50 minutes)
This part of the exam aims to assess real world decision making. You are given 10 minutes to study some clinical data, usually a case history with biochemical and haematological test results, an ECG and a chest X-ray.

You then spend 20 minutes discussing this material with an examiner.

Finally you will spend another 20 minutes with a second examiner discussing several unrelated clinical scenarios.

The long case is usually a 'grey' clinical problem. You will be offered a patient who has significant co-morbidities, some of which may be undiagnosed but suggested from the information given. They will not have had a full set of relevant investigations, but they will listed for a procedure that will probably have to be done at some point soon because it is an emergency or a tumour.

You should presume you are working in a good DGH. You will be able to get a cardiac echo on the same day, but a stress echo will probably take a week, the wards will be able to manage epidural analgesia and there will always be an ITU bed if you need it.

The first question asked is always 'please summarise the case'. Use the time available at the start to try to pull the information offered together into a coherent story, of 4 or 5 punchy sentences. You will then move on to talk about the history, the investigations, and will be asked if you think you need any other investigations. No matter how sick your patient is, and how much you protest, the examiners will eventually force you to 'give an anaesthetic'. Expect this and be prepared, including calculating tube sizes and drug doses for a paediatric case (it is surprisingly hard to do mental arithmetic when faced by the examiners). Do not forget to plan for the patient's destination after their operation (it is invariably going to be ITU/HDU).

Viva 2 – The Basic Sciences Viva (30 minutes)
This viva is intended to focus on intensive care, pain management and the application of basic sciences to these disciplines. Many of the topics are straight out of the Primary FRCA syllabus. There are two examiners and you will spend 15 minutes with each of them.

How To Use This Book
This book contains four complete SAQ papers, four MCQ papers and four mock vivas. All of the questions are designed to be very similar to those likely to be encountered in the examination.

People who are in their thirties and who have been passing exams every year since they were sixteen do not really need to be told how to revise. We hope that candidates look at the breadth and depth of questions in this book to help them plan their revision. But we hope that this book will find most use in the month before the exam, when all the hard work has been done, to enable realistic practice of both the written papers, and working with a partner the vivas, to hone examination technique.

There is no substitute for a sound knowledge base and no candidate can pass the examination without this. However, an understanding of the structure of the exam and plenty of practice on MCQs, SAQs and vivas will increase your chances of success.

Prepare well!

Sarah Chieveley-Williams
James Holding
Tim Isitt

Abbreviations

ADH	Antidiuretic hormone
APTT	Activated partial thromboplastin time
ARDS	Acute respiratory distress syndrome
ASD	Atrial septal defect
ATN	Acute tubular necrosis
CCF	Congestive cardiac failure
CO	Carbon monoxide
CPAP	Continuous positive airway pressure
CVP	Central venous pressure
DDAVP	Desmopressin
DIC	Disseminated intravascular coagulation
DVT	Deep vein thrombosis
EDRF	Endothelin derived relaxant factor
EMD	Electromechanical dissociation
ETT	Endotracheal tube
FFP	Fresh frozen plasma
FGF	Fresh gas flow
FRC	Functional residual capacity
GCS	Glasgow coma scale
GTN	Glyceryl trinitrate
HDU	High dependency unit
HELLP	Haemolysis, elevated liver function tests and low platelets
HOCM	Hypertrophic obstructive cardiomyopathy
HRT	Hormone replacement therapy
IAP	Intra-abdominal pressure
INF	International normalised ratio
IOP	Intraocular pressure
JVP	Jugular venous pressure
LVF	Left ventricular failure
MAOIs	Monoamine oxidase inhibitors
MAC	Minimum alveolar concentration
MCV	Mean corpuscular volume
MDMA	Ecstasy
MH	Malignant hyperpyrexia
N2O	Nitrous oxide
NMDA	N-methyl-D-aspartate
NSAIDs	Non-steroidal anti-inflammatory drugs

OCP	Oral contraceptive pill
PAOP	Pulmonary artery occlusive pressure
PCA	Patient controlled analgesia
PDA	Patent ductus arteriosus
PDPH	Post dural puncture headache
PE	Pulmonary embolus
PEA	Pulseless electrical activity
PEEP	Positive end expiratory pressure
PEFR	Peak expiratory flow rate
PT	Prothrombin time
SIADH	Syndrome of inappropriate antidiuretic hormone
rTPA	Recombinant tissue plasminogen activator
TLCO	Carbon monoxide transfer factor
TPN	Total parenteral nutrition
TV	Tidal volume
VSD	Ventricular septal defect

Recommended Reading List

There are many excellent textbooks on the market. Listed below are the books I found personally of great use for the Final FRCA examination.

A-Z of Anaesthesia: Yentis S, Hirsch N P and Smith G P, 3rd edition, Butterworth Heinemann 2003.

Clinical Textbook of Anaesthesia: Aitkinhead A R and Jones R M, 5th revision Churchill Livingstone 2006.

Acute Medicine Algorithm: Singer M and Webb A, Oxford University Press 1994.

Essays and MCQs in Anaesthesia and Intensive Care: Murphy P M, Edward Arnold 1994.

Handbook of Clinical Anaesthesia: Goldstone J C and Pollard B J, 2nd edition Churchill Livingstone 2003.

Intensive Care: Hinds C J, 2nd edition, Ballière Tindall 1995.

Key Topics in Anaesthesia: Craft T and Upton P, 3rd edition, Bios 2001.

Numerous journals are available, listed below are some that I found very useful:

Anesthesiology

Anaesthesia

British Journal of Anaesthesia - editorials and reviews are often very good

British Journal of Hospital Medicine

British Medical Journal

Continuing education in anaesthesia,critical care and pain (free with BJA)

Current Anaesthesia and Critical Care

Current Opinions in Anaesthesiology

Recommended Reading List

Websites

www.rcoa.ac.uk Royal College of Anaesthetists

www.frca.co.uk Tutorials and past questions

Short Answer Question Paper 1

1. List the principal differential diagnoses of acute stridor in a 3-year-old child (40%). Outline the management of life-threatening epiglottitis in a 3-year-old child. (60%)

2. A 40-year-old man is admitted with an acute head injury. List the indications for intubation and mechanical ventilation. (60%) What are the indications for referral to a neurosurgical unit? (40%)

3. Design a protocol for the management of massive intra-partum haemorrhage.

4. What information about benefits (30%) and side-effects (70%) do you give to a pregnant woman requesting epidural analgesia for relief of labour pain?

5. What investigations are available to preoperatively evaluate the patient with known cardiac ischaemia? (60%) Comment on the usefulness of each test.(40%)

6. Outline, with reasons, the management in the A&E Department of an elderly patient who has been found collapsed at home next to a faulty gas heater.

7. Outline your management of an adult patient brought into the A&E Department in status asthmaticus.

8. What is patient-controlled analgesia (PCA)? (20%) What are the advantages and disadvantages of PCA for postoperative pain control? (80%)

9. Describe the principles behind the capnograph (20%). What information can be obtained from this piece of monitoring equipment? (80%)

10. List the main complications that may occur during transurethral resection of the prostate (TURP). (60%) How would you treat a patient who is confused following TURP? (40%)

11. How would you investigate a patient who has had a severe allergic reaction during anaesthesia? (60%) What are the common causes of life-threatening allergic reactions during anaesthesia? (40%)

12. Summarise the causes (20%), effects (20%) and prevention (60%) of aspiration pneumonitis.

Multiple Choice Question Paper 1

1 The following are statistical tests suitable for ordinal data

❑ A unpaired *t*-test
❑ B Mann–Whitney rank-sum test
❑ C Wilcoxon signed-rank test
❑ D repeated-measures ANOVA
❑ E Pearson's coefficient of linear correlation

2 Spirometry results that give a normal FVC but a reduced FEV_1 could be caused by

❑ A asthma
❑ B laryngeal tumour
❑ C pulmonary oedema
❑ D lung fibrosis
❑ E post pneumonectomy

3 Ultrasound guidance for central venous access

❑ A is the technique recommended by the National Institute of Health and Clinical Excellence
❑ B removes the risk of iatrogenic pneumothorax
❑ C fluid in vessels shows up as bright (white) on the screen
❑ D is ideal for subclavian vein cannulation
❑ E a specially formulated gel must be used between probe and skin

4 Decontamination of flexible fibreoptic laryngoscopes

❑ A before decontamination the scope should be leak tested
❑ B the first stage involves cleaning in enzymatic detergent
❑ C glutaraldehyde is a suitable agent for chemical high level disinfection
❑ D electrolysed saline (eg Sterilox) is a suitable agent for chemical high level disinfection
❑ E autoclaving is an alternative to chemical high level disinfection

5 In the ECG

❑ A the T wave represents ventricular depolarisation
❑ B K^+ is the major ion causing the transmembrane potential
❑ C the QRS duration depends on the recording electrode
❑ D a recording of V_1 needs two sensing electrodes
❑ E a positive deflection occurs when depolarisation is going away from the recording electrode

6 Wright's respirometer

❑ A is inaccurate at flows of <1 l/min
❑ B is a turbine
❑ C is affected by the viscosity of gas
❑ D is affected by humidity
❑ E can be used to measure peak flow

7 The advantages of SIMV over CMV include

❑ A better ventilatory gas distribution
❑ B lower mean airway pressures
❑ C less haemodynamic disturbance
❑ D better matching of ventilation to metabolic demand
❑ E reduced muscle work

8 The following are the units of fundamental (as opposed to derived) physical phenomena

❑ A kilogram
❑ B second
❑ C volt
❑ D pascal
❑ E candela

9 Laminar flow through a tube

❑ A is proportional to the pressure gradient
❑ B is proportional to the viscosity
❑ C is inversely proportional to the density
❑ D is proportional to the tube diameter to the power of four
❑ E may become turbulent if the velocity decreases

10 Diathermy

- ❑ A unipolar diathermy delivers direct current between two electrodes
- ❑ B bipolar diathermy utilises low-frequency alternating current
- ❑ C the device often contains a capacitor in series to act as a filter
- ❑ D to avoid interference the earth plate is placed away from metal prostheses
- ❑ E may cause ignition of alcohol skin prep

11 Concerning bilirubin metabolism

- ❑ A the diglucuronide is mostly formed in the liver
- ❑ B prior phenobarbitone treatment leads to enhanced conjugation
- ❑ C unconjugated bilirubin is damaging to the neonate
- ❑ D in haemolysis the bilirubin is mostly unconjugated
- ❑ E in extra-hepatic obstructive jaundice the bilirubin is mostly conjugated

12 Pulmonary oedema is seen in

- ❑ A aortic stenosis
- ❑ B left atrial myxoma
- ❑ C massive pulmonary embolus
- ❑ D mitral stenosis
- ❑ E tricuspid stenosis

13 The following are seen in chronic renal failure

- ❑ A hypercalcaemia
- ❑ B hyponatraemia
- ❑ C hyperkalaemia
- ❑ D hypoproteinaemia
- ❑ E microcytic anaemia

14 In haemophilia A

- ❑ A there is a prolonged prothrombin time
- ❑ B there is polyarthropathy
- ❑ C gastrointestinal haemorrhage occurs
- ❑ D there is a deficiency of factor VIII
- ❑ E DDAVP may be given therapeutically

15 Problems in Crohn's disease include

- ❑ A polyarthropathy
- ❑ B fistula in ano
- ❑ C entero-enteric fistulae
- ❑ D lymphoma
- ❑ E recurrence at operation site

16 Hypotension following removal of a phaeochromocytoma may be due to

- ❑ A acute adrenal failure
- ❑ B reduced intravascular volume
- ❑ C myocardial infarction
- ❑ D retroperitoneal haemorrhage
- ❑ E sepsis

17 Characteristics of acute tubular necrosis are

- ❑ A malignant hypertension
- ❑ B a raised plasma urea but normal creatinine
- ❑ C concentrated urine
- ❑ D hyperkalaemia
- ❑ E a rapidly rising CVP

18 Immediate problems following thyroidectomy include

- ❑ A hypocalcaemia
- ❑ B tracheal collapse
- ❑ C persistent laryngeal stridor
- ❑ D thyroid crisis
- ❑ E respiratory obstruction

19 Extrapyramidal side-effects are seen with

- ❑ A chlorpropamide
- ❑ B carbimazole
- ❑ C droperidol
- ❑ D metoclopramide
- ❑ E perphenazine

20 Propranolol

❑ A causes hyperglycaemia
❑ B causes reduced airway resistance
❑ C is contraindicated with verapamil
❑ D is the treatment of choice for post MI ventricular ectopics
❑ E causes selective blockade of beta-1 adrenergic receptors

21 Features of Down's syndrome include

❑ A atrial septal defect
❑ B trisomy 21
❑ C acute leukaemia
❑ D webbed neck
❑ E mental impairment

22 Medical complications of bronchial carcinoma include

❑ A peripheral neuropathy developing before diagnosis of the cancer
❑ B a common occurrence is lymphocytic meningitis
❑ C cerebellar degeneration without evidence of metastases
❑ D hypertrophic pulmonary osteoarthropathy
❑ E Horner's syndrome

23 A fixed, low cardiac output occurs in

❑ A Paget's disease
❑ B Eisenmenger's syndrome
❑ C constrictive pericarditis
❑ D anaemia
❑ E aortic stenosis

24 A 'pink puffer', when compared with a 'blue bloater', will have

❑ A cor pulmonale
❑ B reduced sensitivity to respiratory drive from CO_2
❑ C a higher haematocrit
❑ D a lower P_aO_2
❑ E a lower P_aCO_2

25 Peak flow

- ❑ A is not effort dependent
- ❑ B is measured by pneumotachograph
- ❑ C is measured by vitalograph
- ❑ D is reduced in acute asthma
- ❑ E has diurnal variation

26 Glycosuria occurs in

- ❑ A pregnancy
- ❑ B partial gastrectomy
- ❑ C head injury
- ❑ D phaeochromocytoma
- ❑ E acromegaly

27 Chronic renal failure is associated with

- ❑ A microcytic hypochromic anaemia
- ❑ B hypertension
- ❑ C bleeding disorder
- ❑ D a right shift of the oxygen–haemoglobin dissociation curve
- ❑ E secondary hyperparathyroidism

28 Thrombolytic therapy

- ❑ A is best accomplished with rt-PA
- ❑ B is associated with malignant ventricular dysrhythmias
- ❑ C should be combined with aspirin
- ❑ D can safely be performed within 24 h of major surgery
- ❑ E cannot be repeated within 3 months with streptokinase

29 In aortic regurgitation

- ❑ A angina only occurs when there is coexistent coronary atheroma
- ❑ B there is always a systolic pressure gradient across the aortic valve
- ❑ C the murmur is best heard in the left lateral position
- ❑ D the stroke volume is three times normal
- ❑ E there is typically a diastolic thrill

30 Pulmonary fibrosis may occur with

- ❑ A bleomycin
- ❑ B paraquat
- ❑ C beryllium
- ❑ D cortisone hemisuccinate
- ❑ E amiodarone

31 Platelet administration

- ❑ A needs filtration
- ❑ B needs cross-matching
- ❑ C causes significant increase in plasma histamine
- ❑ D contains citrate
- ❑ E platelets are viable after 2 weeks' storage

32 In effective basic life support during resuscitation

- ❑ A the inspired oxygen is 14%
- ❑ B the expired carbon dioxide is 2%
- ❑ C the pH of arterial blood should be >7.4
- ❑ D the mixed venous oxygen saturation should be >75%
- ❑ E the systolic blood pressure should be >100 mmHg

33 Glutamine

- ❑ A is an essential amino acid
- ❑ B is a nutrient for enterocytes
- ❑ C is a nutrient for polymorphonuclear leucocytes
- ❑ D may be incorporated into total parenteral nutrition
- ❑ E allergy causes coeliac disease

34 Severe salicylate poisoning causes

- ❑ A thrombocytopenia
- ❑ B hypoprothrombinaemia
- ❑ C hypofibrinogenaemia
- ❑ D haemolysis
- ❑ E metabolic acidosis

35 The following occur in acute respiratory distress syndrome (ARDS)

❑ A decreased P_aO_2
❑ B decreased P_aCO_2
❑ C reduced lung compliance
❑ D reduced airway resistance
❑ E reduced diffusion capacity

36 The immediate treatment of anaphylaxis involves

❑ A adrenaline
❑ B ephedrine
❑ C chlorpheniramine
❑ D hydrocortisone
❑ E 0.9% saline

37 Nitric oxide

❑ A is a bronchodilator
❑ B is synthesised from aspartamine
❑ C shows tachyphylaxis
❑ D is used therapeutically in a dose of 10–100 ppm
❑ E has an extremely high affinity for haemoglobin

38 Pulmonary artery occlusive pressure is a good guide to left ventricular end-diastolic volume in

❑ A cardiomyopathy
❑ B mitral stenosis
❑ C aortic incompetence
❑ D pulmonary stenosis
❑ E myocardial infarction

39 Variables used in the APACHE III score include

❑ A toe temperature
❑ B gastric blood flow
❑ C haematocrit
❑ D response to dobutamine
❑ E age of the patient

40 Endotoxin

- ❑ A is always found in septic patients
- ❑ B the test for its presence depends on crab's blood
- ❑ C a treatment for sepsis used antibody to the O antigen of endotoxin
- ❑ D may cause systemic hypotension
- ❑ E may cause pulmonary hypertension

41 In a patient with a flail chest, being ventilated, losing 1.5 l/min, treatment should include

- ❑ A reducing fresh gas flow by 1.5 l/min
- ❑ B adding 10 cm positive end-expiratory pressure
- ❑ C reducing the peak inspiratory flow rate
- ❑ D increasing fresh gas flow by 1.5 l/min
- ❑ E inserting a chest drain

42 In paracetamol poisoning

- ❑ A N-acetylcysteine is a useful treatment
- ❑ B methionine is a useful treatment
- ❑ C jaundice is an early sign
- ❑ D prothrombin time is of prognostic value
- ❑ E liver transplant may be required

43 A patient is likely to be successfully weaned from mechanical ventilation if

- ❑ A they are deeply sedated
- ❑ B they require an inspired oxygen concentration of 60%
- ❑ C the magnitude of Pimax is > –30 cmH_2O
- ❑ D their chest X-ray shows pulmonary oedema
- ❑ E they are acidotic

44 The following have been employed in the treatment of ARDS

- ❑ A kinetotherapy
- ❑ B nitric oxide
- ❑ C nebulised prostacyclin
- ❑ D high frequency jet ventilation
- ❑ E IVOX

45 Concerning tetanus

- ❑ A Tetnolysin, a toxin produced by *Clostridium tetani*, is responsible for the clinical manifestations of tetanus
- ❑ B The toxin causes inhibition of acetylcholine release from lower motor neurones and resultant rigidity
- ❑ C In the early stages of tetanus the patient's life is most at risk from laryngeal and respiratory muscle spasm
- ❑ D Mortality is more than 90% for those admitted to ITU
- ❑ E Natural infection confers life-long immunity

46 The following support the diagnosis of fat embolism syndrome

- ❑ A petechial rash over the thighs and buttocks
- ❑ B acute hypoxaemia P_aO_2 <8 kPa
- ❑ C unexpected neurological signs
- ❑ D elevated serum lipase
- ❑ E electrocardiographic signs of left heart strain

47 Concerning high-frequency jet ventilation (HFJV)

- ❑ A the tidal volume is usually less than the anatomical dead space
- ❑ B it operates at frequencies of 60–600 breaths per minute
- ❑ C the expiratory phase is active
- ❑ D it is used following tracheal repair so that ventilation may be achieved with low mean airway pressures
- ❑ E it allows physiotherapy and airway toilet to be achieved without disconnection and subsequent lung de-recruitment

48 Concerning weakness associated with ICU care

- ❑ A Critical illness polyneuropathy affects both motor and sensory fibres
- ❑ B Acute inflammatory demyelinating polyneuropathy is commonly precipitated by SIRS
- ❑ C The creatinine phosphokinase is markedly elevated in critical illness polyneuropathy
- ❑ D Thick filament myopathy is associated with asthma, steroids and neuromuscular blocking drugs
- ❑ E Necrotising myopathy of intensive care is the commonest cause of weakness in ICU

49 Causes of pulmonary hypertension include

❑ A increased pulmonary venous pressure due to pulmonary stenosis
❑ B pulmonary vasoconstriction due to hypoxia
❑ C pulmonary vascular obstruction due to a patent ductus arteriosus
❑ D pulmonary vasoconstriction following inhalation of epoprostenol
❑ E increased pulmonary blood flow from a ventricular septal defect

50 Concerning catheter-related blood stream infections (CR-BSI)

❑ A the commonest infective organism is streptococcus
❑ B microbiological diagnosis can be made using the differential time to positivity of blood cultures taken simultaneously from the catheter and a peripheral vein
❑ C of catheters removed on the basis of fever and leucocytosis over 80% will be infected
❑ D endoluminal brush sampling is the method of choice for microbiological diagnosis
❑ E anti-microbial impregnated CVCs are effective in reducing CR-BSI

51 Trigeminal neuralgia

❑ A involves the 7th cranial nerve
❑ B is treated with radiofrequency ablation
❑ C is treated with glycerol injection
❑ D produces motor paralysis
❑ E is treated with carbamazepine

52 Halothane

❑ A initially causes a reduction in respiratory rate
❑ B inhibits hypoxic pulmonary vasoconstriction
❑ C inhibits baroreceptors
❑ D is a bronchodilator
❑ E may cause a nodal bradycardia

53 When compared with fentanyl, alfentanil

❑ A has a greater volume of distribution
❑ B is more potent
❑ C has a faster onset of action
❑ D is more protein bound
❑ E has a longer elimination half-life

54 The following drugs are metabolised by cholinesterase

- ❑ A mivacurium
- ❑ B esmolol
- ❑ C cocaine
- ❑ D bupivacaine
- ❑ E aspirin

55 The following drugs are effective transdermally

- ❑ A morphine
- ❑ B fentanyl
- ❑ C atropine
- ❑ D hyoscine
- ❑ E glyceryl trinitrate (GTN)

56 A patient whose blood group is O Rh –ve has

- ❑ A anti-A agglutinin
- ❑ B anti-B agglutinin
- ❑ C anti-Rh agglutinin
- ❑ D anti-Kell antibodies
- ❑ E A and B agglutinogens

57 A young Afro-Caribbean boy needs open reduction and internal fixation of a fractured tibia. His Hb is 7.9 g/dl despite minimal blood loss. He should have

- ❑ A a Sickledex test
- ❑ B transfusion of blood to a Hb of 10 g/dl pre-op
- ❑ C a perioperative bicarbonate infusion
- ❑ D hypotensive anaesthesia
- ❑ E cold intravenous fluids

58 Hypotension during spinal anaesthesia may be caused by

- ❑ A bradycardia
- ❑ B autonomic blockade
- ❑ C hypovolaemia
- ❑ D aortocaval compression
- ❑ E anxiety

59 Normal values for a 3.5 kg neonate are:

- ❑ A a tidal volume of 60 ml
- ❑ B a blood volume of 500 ml
- ❑ C anatomical dead space of 2 ml/kg
- ❑ D a Hb of 17 g/dl
- ❑ E a cardiac output of 1.5 l/min

60 Stellate ganglion block produces

- ❑ A mydriasis
- ❑ B postural hypotension
- ❑ C vasodilatation in the ipsilateral arm
- ❑ D reduced lacrimation
- ❑ E loss of the consensual light reflex

61 Postoperative hypertension is commonly due to

- ❑ A pain
- ❑ B hypocapnia
- ❑ C a full bladder
- ❑ D the residual effects of inhalation agents
- ❑ E phaeochromocytoma

62 You are called urgently to the labour ward by the obstetrician who has administered ergometrine. The uterus has contracted down and he cannot extract the second twin. The effects can be reversed by

- ❑ A isoflurane
- ❑ B thiopentone
- ❑ C salbutamol
- ❑ D ritodrine
- ❑ E suxamethonium

63 Suxamethonium is contraindicated in

- ❑ A dystrophia myotonica
- ❑ B acute intermittent porphyria
- ❑ C sickle cell disease
- ❑ D the neonate
- ❑ E congestive cardiac failure

64 Problems associated with laparoscopic surgery include

- ❑ A increased risk of regurgitation
- ❑ B gas embolism
- ❑ C pneumothorax
- ❑ D arrhythmias
- ❑ E shoulder tip pain

65 In total hip replacement

- ❑ A non-steroidal anti-inflammatory drugs may precipitate acute renal failure
- ❑ B regional techniques reduce long-term mortality
- ❑ C hypoxia intra-operatively may be due to embolism
- ❑ D hyperventilation is beneficial
- ❑ E methyl methacrylate is positively inotropic

66 The following nerves may be damaged in the lithotomy position

- ❑ A common peroneal
- ❑ B femoral
- ❑ C obturator
- ❑ D saphenous
- ❑ E lateral cutaneous nerve of the thigh

67 The tachycardia produced by isoprenaline may be blocked by

- ❑ A atropine
- ❑ B nifedipine
- ❑ C phenobarbitone
- ❑ D propranolol
- ❑ E trimetaphan

68 Hepatitis B may be transmitted by

- ❑ A platelets
- ❑ B fibrinogen
- ❑ C albumin
- ❑ D plasma
- ❑ E packed red cells

69 The femoral nerve

- ❑ A lies outside the femoral sheath
- ❑ B lies medial to the femoral artery
- ❑ C gives a cutaneous branch to the scrotum
- ❑ D is blocked in a '3:1' block
- ❑ E is suitably blocked for foot surgery

70 Side-effects of amiodarone are

- ❑ A hypothyroidism
- ❑ B photosensitivity
- ❑ C corneal micro-deposits
- ❑ D peripheral neuropathy
- ❑ E pulmonary fibrosis

71 A spinal block is relatively contraindicated in

- ❑ A placenta praevia
- ❑ B pre-eclampsia
- ❑ C hypovolaemia
- ❑ D breech presentation
- ❑ E fetal distress

72 A tourniquet is applied to the leg for two hours. Signs of nerve damage include

- ❑ A extensor plantar
- ❑ B ankle clonus
- ❑ C reduced vibration sense at the ankle
- ❑ D reduced pin prick at the toe
- ❑ E reduced movement at the ankle after stimulation of the common peroneal nerve

73 A patient who takes a monoamine oxidase inhibitor suddenly develops a BP of 230/130 mmHg after being given ephedrine. Suitable treatment includes

- ❑ A labetalol
- ❑ B propranolol
- ❑ C phenobarbitone
- ❑ D diazoxide
- ❑ E guanethidine

74 Epidural anaesthesia is associated with the following

- ❑ A an increased rate of instrumental delivery
- ❑ B headache
- ❑ C backache
- ❑ D urinary retention
- ❑ E deep vein thrombosis

75 The following suggest inadequate perfusion in posterior fossa surgery

- ❑ A delta waves on EEG
- ❑ B arrhythmias
- ❑ C rise in BP
- ❑ D decrease in temperature
- ❑ E abnormal respiratory pattern

76 Propofol

- ❑ A produces green urine as a side-effect
- ❑ B causes less cardiac depression than thiopentone
- ❑ C is solubilised in egg phosphatide and glycerol emulsion
- ❑ D is 2,6 di-isopropyl phenol
- ❑ E is metabolised only in the liver

77 Nitrous oxide

- ❑ A is contraindicated in tympanoplasty
- ❑ B causes vitamin B_{12} deficiency
- ❑ C inhibits folate metabolism
- ❑ D is stored as a gas
- ❑ E is stored in blue cylinders

78 Morbid obesity is associated with

- ❑ A reduced incidence of difficult intubation
- ❑ B an increased risk of regurgitation of acidic gastric contents
- ❑ C increased chest compliance
- ❑ D increased airways resistance
- ❑ E increased hypoxaemia during general anaesthesia

79 A supraclavicular brachial plexus block is more likely than an axillary block to produce

- ❑ A analgesia of shoulder
- ❑ B analgesia of fingers
- ❑ C a pneumothorax
- ❑ D intravascular injection
- ❑ E a Horner's syndrome

80 In the autonomic nervous system

- ❑ A acetylcholine is the neurotransmitter at all ganglia
- ❑ B noradrenaline is the neurotransmitter at postganglionic sympathetic nerves
- ❑ C relaxation of the uterus is mediated by beta- 2 adrenoreceptors
- ❑ D beta adrenergic receptors are linked to adenylate cyclase
- ❑ E the action of noradrenaline is terminated mainly by metabolism

81 The following are appropriate analgesic doses for an 8-kg baby

- ❑ A Paracetamol PO 160 mg QDS
- ❑ B Diclofenac PR 25 mg TDS
- ❑ C Ibuprofen PO 200 mg TDS
- ❑ D Morphine IV bolus 0.8 mg
- ❑ E Codeine IM 24 mg QDS

82 Gabapentin

- ❑ A is an antagonist at the GABA receptor
- ❑ B is an agonist at the GABA receptor
- ❑ C may modulate NMDA receptors
- ❑ D is an anticonvulsant
- ❑ E is used to treat neuropathic pain

83 Definitions

- ❑ A allodynia – perception of an ordinary non-noxious stimulus as painful
- ❑ B dysaesthesia – pain in an area that lacks sensation
- ❑ C paraesthesia – pain in the distribution of a nerve or group of nerves
- ❑ D hyperaesthesia – increased response to mild stimulation
- ❑ E radiculopathy – functional abnormality of one or more nerve roots

84 Carcinoid syndrome

- ❑ A the classic syndrome is of diarrhoea, flushing, hypotension, and bronchospasm
- ❑ B hypertension can occur
- ❑ C endocardial fibrosis tends to involve the aortic and mitral valves
- ❑ D 5-hydroxytryptamine (5HT) is usually the mediator
- ❑ E hyperglycaemia is a feature

85 Congenital heart disease with right to left shunt

- ❑ A inhalational induction takes longer than usual
- ❑ B nitric oxide is used to decrease systemic vascular resistance
- ❑ C where possible neuraxial blocks are the technique of choice
- ❑ D lesions requiring ductus arteriosus patency may require prostaglandin E_1 infusion
- ❑ E intravenous induction takes longer than usual

86 Syringe labelling in critical care areas (2004 guidelines)

- ❑ A induction agents have yellow labels
- ❑ B muscle relaxants have violet labels
- ❑ C anticholinergic agents have green labels
- ❑ D antagonists are denoted with 1-mm-wide diagonal stripes
- ❑ E the labels for suxamethonium and adrenaline are different from the others

87 Consent for anaesthesia

- ❑ A elective patients should receive written information about anaesthesia before they meet their anaesthetist
- ❑ B the anaesthetic room is an acceptable place to provide elective patients with new information
- ❑ C a separate formal written consent form should be signed by all patients before awake intubation
- ❑ D patient questions about the safety of the proposed anaesthetic technique should be laughed off
- ❑ E adults should be presumed to have capacity to consent unless there is contrary evidence

88 Day surgery

- ❑ A the NHS plans to perform 75% of elective surgery as day cases
- ❑ B suitability for day surgery is based on age and ASA
- ❑ C central neural blockade can be used for day surgery
- ❑ D audit has no place in day surgery
- ❑ E there is evidence that all patients should receive prophylactic anti-emetics

89 Management of anaesthesia for Jehovah's Witnesses

- ❑ A transfusion of allogeneic blood is specifically forbidden by the religion
- ❑ B transplantation of solid organs is specifically forbidden by the religion
- ❑ C intra-operative blood salvage is specifically forbidden by the religion
- ❑ D an individual anaesthetist may 'opt-out' of having to provide direct care
- ❑ E in a life-threatening emergency in a child unable to give competent consent, all life-saving treatment should be given, irrespective of the parents' wishes

90 The following drugs have anticonvulsant effects

- ❑ A midazolam
- ❑ B morphine
- ❑ C gabapentin
- ❑ D flumazenil
- ❑ E magnesium sulphate

Practice Paper 1: The Clinical Vivas

Viva 1: The Clinical Viva takes place in the morning.

1. You are given a piece of clinical information and you have 10 min to study it.
2. You will spend 20 min with the first examiner, discussing the clinical care of the patient described and how you would anaesthetise for the case.
3. You will then spend 20 min with a second examiner discussing approximately three unrelated clinical scenarios.

Viva 2: The Clinical Science Viva takes place in the afternoon. Two examiners will question you for approximately 15 min each.

Approximately four topics are covered.

A good way to prepare for the viva is to work with a partner. For this reason we have separated the sample questions in this book from the model answers to allow you to work through the viva session before looking at the answers.

Viva 1

Clinical scenario

A 77-year-old lady is admitted for removal of cataract and insertion of an intraocular lens implant. She refuses local anaesthetic.

She suffered a myocardial infarct 9 years ago. She now only suffers infrequent angina for which she has a glyceryl trinitrate spray. Three years ago she had an operation because her right arm became pale, white and mottled.

Her current medications include warfarin, digoxin 0.125 mg mane and Frumil® one daily.

On examination the positive findings are blowing pansystolic and early rumbling diastolic murmurs loudest at the apex. She has an irregularly irregular pulse and fine basal crepitations on auscultation of the lung fields. The apex beat is displaced in the 6th intercostal space in the anterior axillary line.

Her ECG and CXR are shown in Fig. 1 and Fig. 2 respectively.

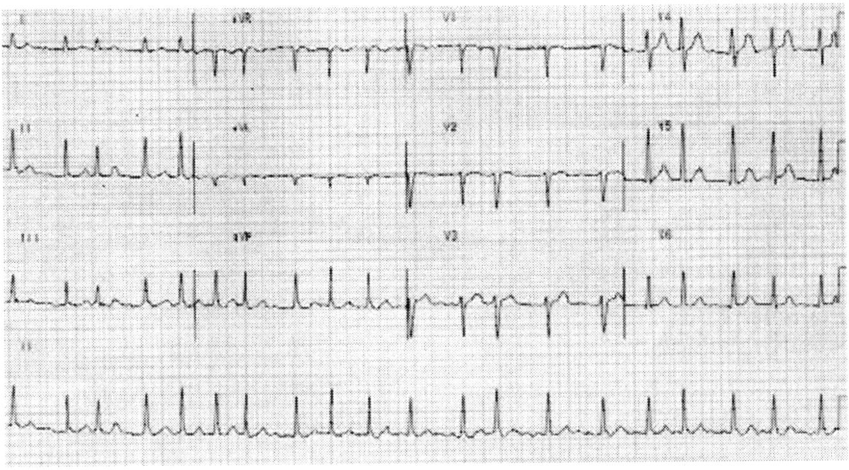

Fig. 1: ECG

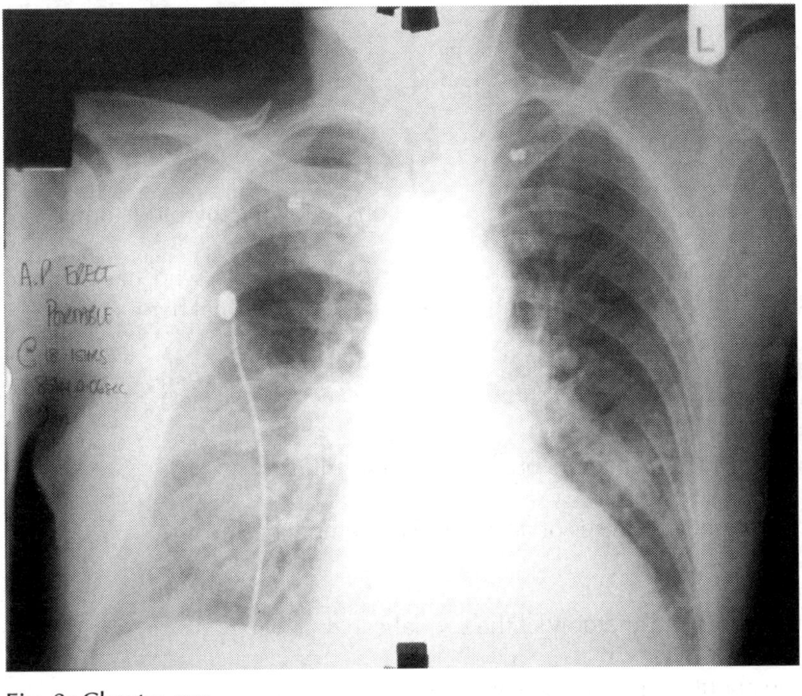

Fig. 2: Chest x-ray

Her biochemistry results are:
Na 140
Glucose 6.2
K 5.5
Urea 10
Creatinine 140
Hb 11.4
WCC 5.8
Pt 256
INR 1.6

Examiner 1
Summarise this lady's case

Tell me about her ECG

Describe the CXR

Describe the cardiac outline, the lung fields and any obvious pathology

How would you anaesthetise this lady?

Examiner 2
Tell me about premedication.

Tell me about the anaesthetic complications following thyroidectomy.

How would you anaesthetise a 25-year-old asthmatic who has a blood pressure of 170/100 mmHg and is due to have an inguinal hernia repair?

Viva 2

Examiner 1
Tell me about the anaemia of chronic renal failure

Tell me about the causes of delayed gastric emptying

Examiner 2
Tell me about the anatomy of the caudal canal

Tell me about the problems of hypotensive anaesthesia

Short Answer Question Paper 1 Answers

1 List the principal differential diagnoses of acute stridor in a 3-year-old child (40%). Outline the management of life-threatening epiglottitis in a 3-year-old child. (60%)

Stridor is a high-pitched inspiratory noise characteristic of upper airway obstruction.

The principal differential diagnoses are:
- Epiglottitis
- Croup
- Inhalation of foreign body
- Diphtheria
- Retropharyngeal abscess/haematoma
- Inhalation injury
- Trauma
- Angioneurotic oedema

Management of epiglottitis:
- Do not upset the child
- No IV access
- No neck X-ray
- Do not change the child's adopted sitting position and do not remove from parents
- Administer humidified oxygen, if feasible
- Call for senior help – anaesthetist/ENT surgeon/paediatrician
- Follow departmental guidelines for management:
  (a) gas induction with oxygen and sevoflurane in a safe environment – theatres/PICU
  (b) minimal monitoring: ECG, oximeter, IV access
  (c) secure airway with ETT when patient deeply anaesthetised – instruments available for tracheostomy
  (d) capnograph to confirm satisfactory intubation
  (e) blood cultures and other investigations to be sent – antibiotics administered – IV fluids given
  (f) sedation for ventilation – pass a nasogastric tube for feeding and oral sedative drugs – admit to ICU bed

2 A 40-year-old man is admitted with an acute head injury. List the indications for intubation and mechanical ventilation. (60%) What are the indications for referral to a neurosurgical unit? (40%)

In a 40-year-old man who has sustained a head injury, the priorities are to avoid hypoxia, hypotension and hypercarbia to prevent secondary brain damage.

The indications for intubation following a head injury:

Immediately

- Coma (not obeying, not speaking, not eye opening), ie a Glasgow Coma Scale (GCS) ≤8
- Loss of protective laryngeal reflexes
- Ventilatory insufficiency (as judged by blood gases):
  - (a) hypoxaemia (P_aO_2 <9 kPa on air or <13 kPa on oxygen)
  - (b) hypercarbia (P_aO_2 >6 kPa)
- Spontaneous hyperventilation causing P_aCO_2 <3.5 kPa
- Respiratory arrhythmias

Before transfer, either inter hospital or intra hospital, eg to CT scanner

- Significantly deteriorating or fluctuating conscious level, even if not in coma
- Bilaterally fractured mandible
- Copious bleeding into mouth (eg from skull base fracture)
- Seizures

All intubated patients must be ventilated with muscle relaxation and appropriate sedation and analgesia. Aim for P_aO_2 >13 kPa, P_aCO_2 4.5–5.0 kPa.

The criteria for referring head-injured patients to a neurosurgical unit:

Immediately (after initial assessment and resuscitation)

- Fractured skull, with any of the following:
  - (a) any alteration of conscious level (GCS <15)
  - (b) focal neurological signs
  - (c) fits
  - (d) any other neurological symptoms/signs
- Coma persisting after resuscitation – even without a skull fracture
- Deterioration of conscious level – even without a skull fracture
- Focal pupil or limb signs – even without a skull fracture
- Abnormal CT scan

Urgently (not necessarily immediately)
- Confusion persisting > 6 h (even without a skull fracture)
- Compound depressed skull fracture (or other penetrating injury)
- Suspected leak of CSF from nose or ear
- Persistent or worsening headache or vomiting (especially in a child)

Ref: Gentleman D, Dearden M, Midgley S, Maclean D. Guidelines for resuscitation and transfer of patients with serious head injury. *Br Med J* 1993; **307**:547–552.

3 Design a protocol for the management of massive intra-partum haemorrhage.

Massive intra-partum haemorrhage is variably defined as more than 1 ml/kg per min blood loss, blood loss >1500 ml, a decrease in haemoglobin >4g/dl or acute transfusion requirement >4 units. The main aim is to initiate resuscitation, to enrol senior help and transfer the patient to theatre as soon as possible.
- If the patient is undelivered, put in left lateral position. Administer oxygen
- Ask for senior anaesthetist/obstetrician/midwife
- Establish IV access with 2×14-G cannulae
- Send bloods at the same time for cross-matching, FBC, clotting
- Inform the blood bank, transfusion haematologist
- Administer colloid with a pressurised giving set
- With every 6 units of blood, give platelets and FFP via a fluid warmer
- Get control of bleeding by going to theatre
- Post-partum haemorrhage may be due to retention of the products of conception. Therefore, consider syntocinon or ergometrine
- Monitor basic parameters: coagulation status, if undelivered the fetal heart rate, and consider direct measurement of central venous pressure and arterial pressure
- Give O-neg blood if cross-matched blood not easily available
- Consider ICU bed for the patient

4 What information about benefits (30%) and side-effects (70%) do you give to a pregnant woman requesting epidural analgesia for relief of labour pain?

The benefits of epidural analgesia
- Analgesia superior to entonox, intramuscular pethidine or TENS

- Easily performed, generally effective with minimal serious side-effects to either mother or fetus
- If necessary can be used for instrumental delivery (forceps, ventouse) or for caesarean section

The commonest side-effects include
- Hypotension, avoided by pre-loading with IV fluid
- Pruritis if opiates are used. Rarely troublesome. Many respond to a small dose of naloxone (40 μg) or propofol (10–20 mg)
- Shivering

These are due to autonomic blockade.
- Dural puncture – occurs in about 1:200 patients. It causes severe headache and may require epidural blood patch.
- Failure of technique – requiring repeat epidural

Less common problems which one may not wish to burden the mother with include
- Urinary retention
- High epidural block
- Inadvertent intravascular injection of local anaesthetic
- Risk of permanent neurological damage – approx 1:14000

It is worth informing the mother that there is an increased chance of her requiring an instrumental delivery with an epidural. The question of whether there is an increased rate of caesarean section after an epidural is sited remains debatable.

Ref: Fetal & Maternal Med Review 1996; **8**:29–55.

5 What investigations are available to preoperatively evaluate the patient with known cardiac ischaemia? (60%) Comment on the usefulness of each test. (40%)

Preoperative investigation of ischaemic heart disease

Standard investigations
- FBC: anaemia, which further compromises coronary oxygen supply, should be excluded
- CXR: a routine CXR should be performed to exclude cardiac failure
- 12-lead ECG: this may be normal or show ST segment or T wave abnormalities indicating ischaemia. Evidence of previous myocardial infarct, rhythm disturbance or conduction abnormality may be present

Specialised investigations

- Exercise stress test: the ECG is continuously monitored while the patient undergoes graded exercise on a treadmill. Although a negative stress test is encouraging it does not exclude coronary artery disease.
- Radionuclear imaging:
  - (a) Thallium scanning: thallium is taken up after intravenous injection by viable myocardium. A fixed defect or 'cold spot' indicates infarcted myocardium whereas reversible defects represent ischaemia.
  - (b) Dipyridamole thallium scanning (DTI): dipyridamole is used to induce coronary vasodilation pharmacologically after which thallium scanning is performed.
  - (c) MUGA scan: the isotope technetium-99 is used. This technique assesses left ventricular ejection fraction, stroke volume and regional wall motion abnormalities.
- Echocardiography: provides information about the heart valves, stroke volume and ejection fraction. It can show areas of dyskinesis and regional wall motion abnormalities due to ischaemic or infarcted myocardium.
- Cardiac catheterisation: although this is an invasive procedure, it remains the gold standard for the demonstration of coronary artery disease.

Ref: Edwards N D and Reilly C S. Detection of perioperative myocardial ischaemia. *Br J Anaesth* 1994; **72**: 104–115.

6 Outline, with reasons, the management in the A&E Department of an elderly patient who has been found collapsed at home next to a faulty gas heater.

Initial management of this patient should involve basic resuscitation – checking the airway (applying a high concentration of oxygen), breathing and circulation. A history should be obtained and the patient examined for associated injuries. The main problem appears to be that of carbon monoxide (CO) poisoning and this should be determined by sending blood not only for FBC, U&E and arterial blood gases but also for CO estimation on a laboratory co-oximeter. Other investigations should include a CXR and ECG.

Carbon monoxide poisoning may present with symptoms of headache and nausea at levels of 15%–20% progressing to coma at levels >40%. CO binds haemoglobin 250 times more avidly than oxygen hence reducing oxygen carriage by the blood. Additionally, it causes a leftward shift of the oxygen dissociation curve and poisons the mitochondrial enzymes, causing a metabolic acidosis.

Measurement is only by a co-oximeter as the IR absorption of CO causes pulse oximeters to read towards 96% saturation.

Treatment involves protection of the airway if the patient is unconscious (GCS < 8) and ventilation with 100% oxygen. This reduces the half-life of CO from 4 h to 45 min. In the unconscious patient, hyperbaric oxygen is also useful but centres with the facility for intermittent positive pressure ventilation (IPPV) in the hyperbaric chamber are rare. Monitoring should include ECG, blood pressure and end-tidal CO_2. The cardiovascular system may require support, and the metabolic acidosis may require management with bicarbonate if severe but this is controversial. Finally, other injuries should be sought and treated appropriately.

7 Outline your management of an adult patient brought into the A&E department in status asthmaticus.

Acute severe asthma (or status asthmaticus) is a medical emergency.

Clinical signs indicating severe attack:
- Inability to speak
- Respiratory rate >25 breaths/min
- Tachycardia >110 beats/min
- P_aO_2 <8 kPa
- P_aCO_2 >6.5 kPa

Particularly ominous signs:
- Silent chest on auscultation
- Cyanosis
- Bradycardia, hypotension (<90 mmHg systolic)
- Confusion
- Exhaustion, respiratory rate >50 or <10 breaths/min

Consider ventilation if:
- P_aO_2 <8 kPa (despite F_iO_2 ≥0.6)
- P_aCO_2 >6 kPa
- pH <7.3

Prior to transfer to ICU:
- Give highest possible inspired oxygen concentration by mask.

- Insert intravenous cannula; 0.5–1 litre of intravenous fluids as often dehydrated. Intubate (rapid sequence induction) and ventilate.
- Pharmacological treatment:
  (a) Nebulised salbutamol every 2–4 h, 5 mg in 5 ml saline in 100% oxygen. Switch to intravenous salbutamol if no response.
  (b) Nebulised ipratropium bromide every 6 h, 0.5 mg in 5 ml saline in 100% oxygen.
  (c) Intravenous aminophylline
    (i) Loading dose (except in patients on regular oral theophyllines): 5 mg/kg over 15–30 min. Signs of toxicity are hypotension, arrhythmias and convulsions.
    (ii) Maintenance dose 0.5–0.9 mg/kg per hour. Narrow therapeutic index.
  Monitor levels regularly (therapeutic range 10–20 mg/l).
  (d) Consider intravenous ketamine, magnesium sulphate (1.2–2g over 20 minutes) or inhaled isoflurane for resistant bronchospasm.
  (e) Intravenous hydrocortisone 100 mg bolus, repeat every 6 h.
  (f) Antibiotics if signs of infection (purulent sputum, fever, leucocytosis).
  (g) Correct fluid/electrolytes, especially K^+ disturbances
- Further investigations: CXR, ECG, repeat arterial blood gases, FBC including WBC, serum potassium.
- Ventilation:
  (a) aim is to oxygenate adequately
  (b) avoid barotrauma
  (c) permissive hypercapnia
  (d) use prolonged expiratory phase
  (e) physiotherapy to clear secretions

Assess response to therapy:
- Clinically
- Blood gases: P_aO_2 and P_aCO_2
- Airway pressures

8 What is patient-controlled analgesia (PCA)? (20%) What are the advantages and disadvantages of PCA for postoperative pain control? (80%)

PCA is a form of postoperative pain control which has been in use in many hospitals over the last 5–8 years. It involves the intravenous admission of boluses delivered by a syringe pump triggered by the patient. The pump is set up by the anaesthetist, the amount of analgesia timed between boluses (lock-out). The maximum dose in 4 h and the possibility of a background infusion are all set before use. The advantages of this method of postoperative analgesia are numerous. Possibly the most important is the fact that the patient controls his/her own pain relief. Studies have shown that patient satisfaction has increased because of this. A major advantage is that the patient does not have to wait for a nurse to get the drug, check with another nurse and then administer it. The other benefits are that the drug is delivered intravenously as opposed to intramuscularly, and small and regular boluses are given as opposed to large infrequent doses, thus leading to a more constant plasma level and implicit safety. Safety is important. The patients control their own level of analgesia and if they are sleepy they will not press the button; therefore, if used correctly, overdoses are extremely unlikely. Finally, other drugs can be included in the PCA such as anti-emetics to control nausea.

A disadvantage is that there is, of course, a potential for malfunction of the pump and, therefore, the delivery of a potentially fatal dose of opiate to the patient. The syringe pump should be attached to the patient by a specialised giving set which has an anti-siphon valve and a one-way valve so that if an intravenous infusion is connected to the patient there can be no risk of the narcotic backing up into the intravenous set.

On the practical side, the button may be difficult to press if the patient has had hand or arm surgery and does not have the strength to push the button; this is particularly relevant to the elderly. The pumps are not suitable for those who cannot understand how to use them and, therefore, in any patients who are confused or children less than 5–6 years of age. Side-effects of the narcotic are nausea, itching, ileus and hallucinations. Patients are not 'painfree' as with a regional technique. Some patients are unable to understand the need or are reluctant to operate the button. Mobility is restricted because of the pump, drip pole, etc.

In general, this form of analgesia is a major advance in postoperative pain control as long as it is set up correctly and is used correctly by the patient and not by their relatives.

9 Describe the principles behind the capnograph (20%). What information can be obtained from this piece of monitoring equipment? (80%)

The capnograph is used to monitor end-tidal carbon dioxide (ET CO2). It employs the Luft principle, which states that any molecule with two or more different atoms will absorb infra-red radiation. The system comprises an infra-red source, a filter to ensure radiation of desired wavelength is transmitted, a sample chamber and photodetector. The fraction of radiation absorbed is compared with a reference gas, thus regular calibration against a reference gas is necessary. The result is then displayed against time to produce a capnogram.

The following information can be obtained:

- Respiratory rate.
- Adequacy of ventilation; the ET CO_2 approximates to P_aCO_2 which provides an assessment of the adequacy of ventilation. Hypoventilation causes a raised ET CO_2, hyperventilation a reduced ET CO_2.
- Indirect assessment of cardiac output; the presence of expired CO_2 (ET CO_2) depends on adequate lung perfusion which in turn depends on the cardiac output. In low cardiac output states the ET CO_2 will be low. In cardiac arrest there is no capnograph trace.
- Disconnection alarm; in event of disconnection of the breathing system/ventilator the capnograph trace will disappear.
- Confirmation of correct placement of the endotracheal tube.
- Detection of malignant hyperpyrexia or other hypermetabolic state, with rising CO_2.
- Detection of pulmonary embolus producing a sudden decline in ET CO_2 (in conjunction with desaturation and hypotension).
- Indirect assessment of neuromuscular block. In the absence of a peripheral nerve stimulator, the capnograph trace may indicate when the neuromuscular block wears off and the patient tries to breathe.
- Detection of re-breathing of carbon dioxide in, for example, inadequate fresh gas flow or exhausted soda lime in a circle system.
- Detection of bronchospasm; the capnograph is altered in patients with chronic airflow limitation and also if bronchospasm develops intra-operatively.

10 List the main complications that may occur during transurethral resection of the prostate (TURP). (60%) How would you treat a patient who is confused following TURP? (40%)

Complications that occur during transurethral resection of the prostate (TURP) may be general (ie those of an elderly population undergoing anaesthesia and surgery) or specific to that operation.

General

- *Cardiovascular*. These elderly patients are at an increased risk of CVS morbidity and mortality. Ischaemia, myocardial infarction, hypotension and arrhythmias may all be encountered.
- *Respiratory*. Pulmonary aspiration is always a potential risk. Chronic pulmonary disease is also relatively common in this population and this may be exacerbated by lithotomy position. Regional anaesthesia may reduce this risk.
- *Other*. There may be deterioration in renal function particularly on a background of chronic renal impairment. Neurological problems may arise ranging from confusion to cerebral infarction.

Specific

- *TUR syndrome*. This is a clinical syndrome of confusion, cardiovascular instability (hypertension, hypotension, arrhythmias, pulmonary oedema) and subsequent unconsciousness and seizure activity.
- *Bladder rupture*. Presents as abdominal pain. Shock and features of excessive water absorption may follow.
- *Bleeding*. This may be excessive both because of excessive gland vascularity and release of fibrinolytic substances such as urokinase.
- *Sepsis*. Bacteraemia may result from the instrumentation of a chronically infected urinary tract.

The differential diagnosis of patient who is confused post TURP includes:

- TUR syndrome
- Other metabolic disturbance such as hypoglycaemia or severe hypoxia
- Neurological event; TIA, CVA

Treatment should be along the lines of airway assessment, breathing adequacy with additional oxygen and circulatory assessment. A brief neurological assessment should follow including GCS and any focal neurological signs.

A brief history should be obtained focusing on preoperative status such as diabetes, previous CVA or dementia as well as the intraoperative course including cardiovascular stability, length of procedure and amount of irrigant used.

Basic investigations including blood gas analysis, blood glucose, full blood count and electrolyte estimation as well as ECG and CXR if there is respiratory compromise.

TUR syndrome: The underlying pathophysiology is the absorption of glycine solution used to irrigate the operative field. This is related to the height of the bags, operator skill and duration of the operation. The patient becomes overloaded with water causing the haemodynamic instability. Initially there is hypertension but later there will be hypotension, bradycardia and a low cardiac output state. Hyponatraemia occurs due to natriuresis and this, coupled with the direct toxic effects of glycine, causes cerebral irritation and confusion, progressing to seizures and unconsciousness. Treatment is with hypertonic saline to increase the serum sodium and improve cardiac function. Occasionally furosemide and ventilatory support will be required to treat overt pulmonary oedema.

Ref: Hahn R G. Fluid absorption in endoscopic surgery. *Br J Anaesth* 2006; **96**(1): 8–19.

11. How would you investigate a patient who has had a severe allergic reaction during anaesthesia? (60%) What are the common causes of life-threatening allergic reactions during anaesthesia? (40%)

- No tests have an immediate benefit on management so they must not take priority over resuscitation in the acute phase.
- Testing has two phases: first to confirm anaphylaxis or anaphylactoid reaction as opposed to other causes of the adverse event; secondly, to investigate the causative substance.
- Once the patient is stable blood should be taken to analyse the mast cell tryptase. The rise in tryptase is transient and ideally blood should be taken immediately after the reaction has been treated, and then 1 h and 6–24 h post reaction. The serum samples should be stored at –20°C until they can be sent for analysis.
- Normal plasma tryptase levels are low, and will be increased in anaphylactoid or anaphylactic reactions. The higher the level the more likely anaphylaxis as opposed to anaphylactoid reaction is the cause.
- Investigation of the causative substance should start at the anaesthetic chart together with history of previous drug exposure. The patient should be referred to a regional allergy centre with details of the reaction including the timing of all drugs in relation to the reaction.
- The allergist can then investigate using skin prick testing or by using intradermal testing to various substances implicated. Specific IgE antibodies can be measured in serum, currently this is only available for succinylcholine.
- Once the allergist has fully investigated, the patient should be given a full explanation of the events, given a letter to present to doctors in

the future and encouraged to wear a Medi-Alert bracelet. The reaction should be reported on the 'yellow card' system.

Common causes of allergic reactions during anaesthesia

- Neuromuscular blocking agents; most commonly succinylcholine, also vecuronium and atracurium. There may be cross reactivity: quaternary ammonium compounds are found in many cosmetics and hair products and may cause sensitisation.
- Latex; either to latex proteins or the substances used in the purification process.
- Colloids, induction agents.
- Antibiotics; penicillins most commonly implicated, with 8% cross reactivity with cephalosporins.

12. Summarise the causes (20%), effects (20%) and prevention (60%) of aspiration pneumonitis.

Aspiration pneumonitis is due to pulmonary damage from aspiration of acidic gastric contents.

Factors predisposing to regurgitation

- Full stomach
- Delayed gastric emptying. Anxiety, trauma, obesity, pain, diabetes, alcohol, opioids and anticholinergic drugs
- Reduced lower oesophageal pressure. Hiatus hernia, pregnancy, atropine, opioids

The effects of aspiration

- Mild cases: reduced oxygen saturation, wheezing or coughing
- Severe cases: marked hypoxaemia, respiratory failure and ARDS may develop requiring artificial ventilation

Prevention

Elective surgery

- No solids for 6 h, no clear fluids for 2 h prior to anaesthesia
- Consider awake intubation or regional technique

Emergency surgery – the following may be considered

- Nasogastric tube to drain stomach contents
- H_2 receptor antagonists or protein pump inhibitor to reduce the acidity of gastric contents

- Metoclopramide or cisapride to promote gastric emptying. Metoclopramide also increases lower oesophageal sphincter tone
- Sodium citrate or other non-particulate antacid to reduce the pH of stomach contents
- Preoxygenation and rapid sequence induction – this secures the airway rapidly
- Cricoid pressure – this manoeuvre compresses the oesophagus between cricoid cartilage and vertebrae and prevents onward passage of any regurgitated material
- Extubate the patient only when he or she is fully awake with protective laryngeal reflexes present
- Awake intubation or regional technique if feasible

Ref: *Hospital Update*. Aspiration and its prevention. May 1994.

Multiple Choice Question Paper 1 Answers

1 The following are statistical tests suitable for ordinal data **Answers: B C**

The unpaired *t*-test tests between two population means when the data are continuous and normally distributed; the Mann–Whitney rank sum test is the equivalent for ordinal data. Wilcoxon's test is the ordinal equivalent of the paired *t*-test.

2 Spirometry results that give a normal FVC but a reduced FEV_1 could be caused by **Answers: A B**

A normal FVC but reduced FEV_1 shows an obstructive lung problem. Obstructive spirometry occurs in asthma, chronic obstructive pulmonary disease (COPD), and tumours. A restrictive spirometry has a low FVC but a normal FEV_1/FVC ratio (about 70%), and occurs in chest wall problems, after lung surgery, pulmonary oedema and lung fibrosis.

3 Ultrasound guidance for central venous access **Answer: A**

Ultrasound is recommended for all central line access by NICE, although they concede that in some emergency conditions a landmark technique may be necessary to save time. It does not remove any of the traditional risks of central access, but it may reduce the risk of pneumothorax. Fluid in vessels shows up as dark (black). It is difficult to visualise the subclavian vein (US does not pass through bone, and the subclavian is below the clavicle). The axillary vein can be seen more laterally, but is usually quite deep and difficult to get to. The purpose of the gel is to exclude air from the ultrasound beam. Although special gels are manufactured, any sterile fluid or gel (eg aqua gel) performs the task just as well.

4 Decontamination of flexible fibreoptic laryngoscopes **Answers: A B D**

First the scope is visually inspected for cracks and is then pressure tested for leaks. It is then cleaned in water and enzymatic detergent to remove visible debris. Chemical high level disinfection can be achieved with electrolysed saline (Sterilox), chlorine dioxide (Tristel), or peracetic acid (Steris, Nu-Cidex). Glutaraldehyde used to be used before it was realised how dangerous it was for the staff. Autoclaving is not suitable for flexible laryngoscopes.

5 The ECG **Answers: All false**

In the ECG the P wave represents atrial depolarisation and the T wave ventricular repolarisation. The QRS complex represents ventricular depolarisation. A positive deflection occurs when the depolarisation is going towards the recording electrode. Sodium is the major ion causing the transmembrane potential. The V (chest leads) record the potential difference between one chest electrode and the 'reference' electrode, which is the sum of at least three limb leads. The duration of the QRS complex is constant, no matter which lead it is recorded from.

6 Wright's respirometer **Answers: A B D**

The Wright respirometer, a turbine, measures gas volume (eg tidal or minute volume). It under-reads at <1 l/min and is affected by moisture which causes the pointer to stick. The pneumotachograph measures flow rate (eg peak flow), and is affected by gas viscosity.

7 The advantages of SIMV over CMV **Answers: A B C D**

Advantages – better ventilatory gas distribution, lower mean airway pressures, less haemodynamic disturbance, ability to assess spontaneous breathing activity, reduced sedation requirement, reduced muscle atrophy and hence easier weaning, the ability to allow spontaneous breaths allows better matching of ventilation to metabolic demands.

Disadvantages – more complex ventilator circuit, high airway resistance, inefficient gas flow, increased work of breathing and therefore muscle fatigue.

8 The following are the units of fundamental (as opposed to derived) physical phenomena **Answers: A B E**

The seven fundamental physical units from which all other SI units may be derived are: metre; kilogram; second; ampere; kelvin; mole; and candela (the units of light intensity).

9 Laminar flow through a tube **Answers: A D**

The Hagen-Poiseuille law states that flow rate is proportional to the pressure gradient (*P*/*l*), the fourth power of the tube diameter (d^4) and inversely proportional to the viscosity (η). The density (ρ) is important for turbulent flow, and for predicting whether flow will be laminar or turbulent (Reynold's number). Flow is more likely to be turbulent as the velocity increases.

10 Diathermy **Answers: C E**

Both unipolar and bipolar diathermy use high-frequency (0.5–1 MHz) alternating current; bipolar is low power. A capacitor can filter out low frequencies. High current densities can develop around metal prostheses increasing the risk of accidental tissue burns.

11 Bilirubin metabolism **Answers: A B C D E**

Bilirubin is formed in the liver from the breakdown of redundant red blood cells. Unconjugated bilirubin is initially formed. The neonate may be damaged if unconjugated bilirubin crosses the immature blood–brain barrier, causing kernicterus (damage to the basal ganglia). In haemolysis there is an increase in unconjugated bilirubin and no bile in the urine.

Bilirubin is conjugated in the hepatocytes and excreted in the bile mainly as the diglucuronide. Conjugation is enhanced by phenobarbitone by induction of the hepatic cytochrome P450 enzyme system. Extra-hepatic jaundice is characterised by pale stools and dark urine. The bilirubin is conjugated.

12 Pulmonary oedema **Answers: B D**

Pulmonary oedema occurs when the left atrial pressure is elevated. This may occur in such diverse conditions as mitral stenosis and left atrial myxoma.

13 Chronic renal failure **Answers: A B C D E**

The patient with chronic renal failure is almost invariably anaemic. The anaemia is usually normocytic. The anaemia would only be hypochromic and microcytic if there was associated iron deficiency, due, for example, to chronic occult blood loss. The anaemia of chronic renal failure is due to lack of erythropoietin production by the kidneys. There is often a bleeding tendency due to platelet dysfunction, although the platelet count is often normal. Hypogastrinaemia and peptic ulceration occur.

There is usually hypocalcaemia with associated hyperphosphataemia.

The kidney is responsible for the conversion of 25-hydroxy cholecalciferol (made in the liver) to the active metabolite 1,25-dihydroxycholecalciferol [$1,25(OH)_2D_3$]. The absorption of calcium from the gut requires $1,25(OH)_2D_3$; in its absence hypocalcaemia occurs. Hypocalcaemia leads to secondary hyperparathyroidism, renal osteodystrophy and hypercalcaemia. The serum albumin is reduced if there is nephrotic syndrome. The serum sodium is normal up to the very terminal stage of chronic renal failure.

14 Haemophilia — Answers: B C D E

Haemophilia is an X-linked recessive haemorrhagic disorder. It is due to deficiency of clotting factor number 8 (factor VIII). As factor VIII is part of the intrinsic clotting cascade, the partial thromboplastin time (APTT) is prolonged, while the prothrombin time (PT) is normal. The platelet count is normal.

Clinically, patients often suffer recurrent painful haemarthroses and muscle haematomas. Prolonged bleeding may occur after circumcision or dental extractions. Haematuria and gastrointestinal haemorrhage may occur. The severity of clinical symptoms depends on the level of factor VIII activity.

Haemophiliacs are treated with regular injections of factor VIII. This used to be supplied from heat-treated pooled serum donations, but factor VIII is now made from recombinant DNA technology which prevents the risk of transmission of HIV or hepatitis C. Factor VIII levels can also effectively be raised by the administration of desmopressin (DDAVP) or cryoprecipitate.

15 Crohn's disease — Answers: A B C D E

Crohn's disease is a granulomatous condition of unknown aetiology. It can affect any part of the gastrointestinal tract from mouth to anus, but most commonly affects the terminal ileum. It commonly presents with abdominal pain and diarrhoea. A low-grade fever, weight loss, anaemia, polyarthropathy, uveitis and skin rashes (erythema nodosum and pyoderma gangrenosum) can all occur. Lymphoma may develop in affected bowel.

Fistula in ano and entero-enteric fistulae are not uncommon. Medical treatment includes the use of corticosteroids, azathioprine and sulphasalazine. Surgery is often necessary, but unfortunately recurrence at the site of operation is not unusual.

16 Hypotensionafter removal of a phaeochromocytoma — Answers: A B C D E

Hypotension after removal of a phaeochromocytoma may be due to all the above causes and in addition may be the result of left ventricular dysfunction or haemorrhage.

17 Acute tubular necrosis — Answers: D E

Acute tubular necrosis (ATN) is characterised by:

(a) a high urinary sodium concentration (> 40 mEq/l)
(b) low urinary urea and creatinine concentrations
(c) low urinary osmolality (<350 mosmol/kg).

In other words, in ATN there is loss of renal concentrating ability by the renal tubules. Thus there is production of poor quality urine with a low osmolality. The tubules fail to conserve sodium and fail to excrete urea and creatinine. By contrast, in dehydration and other causes of pre-renal acute renal failure, the urine is concentrated (urinary osmolality >400 mosmol/kg), the urinary sodium is low (< 20 mEq/l), and there is a high urinary urea and creatinine.

In ATN there will also be hyperkalaemia, an elevated plasma urea and creatinine, and there may be a rapidly rising CVP with pulmonary oedema.

18 Immediate problems post-thyroidectomy — Answers: B C D E

Problems in the postoperative period following a thyroidectomy may be immediate or occur once the patient is back on the ward. Amongst the immediate complications is wound haematoma. The surgeon will usually close the thyroidectomy scar with either clips or staples, and the patient is nursed with a set of instruments at the bedside should it be necessary quickly to evacuate a haematoma which otherwise might lead to tracheal compression and respiratory embarrassment.

Another immediate complication that can occur is tracheal collapse.

Hypocalcaemia, due to removal of one or more of the parathyroid glands at surgery, tends to occur in the early postoperative period, but not immediately. Thyroid crisis can occur intra-operatively or at any time in the post-operative period.

Untreated it may result in coma and be fatal. It usually presents with tachycardia, pyrexia, confusion and abdominal pain and requires treatment with beta blockers and anti-thyroid drugs. Laryngeal stridor may occur due to oedema or direct damage to one or both of the recurrent laryngeal nerves.

19 Extrapyramidal side-effects **Answers: C D E**

Any drug that is an antagonist at dopaminergic receptors can produce extrapyramidal side-effects. In this respect perphenazine is one of the drugs most likely to cause problems. Droperidol also commonly causes this side-effect. The range of extrapyramidal side-effects includes Parkinsonism, dystonia (facial grimacing), akathisia (restlessness) and tardive dyskinesia.

Treatment includes withdrawal of the drug, and administration of an antimuscarinic drug such as procyclidine or benztropine.

20 Propranolol **Answer: C**

Propranolol is a non-selective beta blocker, with actions at both beta-1 and beta-2 adrenoceptors. It causes an increase in airways resistance by blockade of beta-2 receptors in the lungs. Beta blockers are contraindicated with verapamil as they are both negative inotropes. In particular, intravenous verapamil can lead to hypotension and asystole if given to a patient on beta blockers. Beta blockers can lead to a small deterioration in glucose tolerance in diabetics, as well as, more importantly, masking the signs of hypoglycaemia. In the non-diabetic, beta blockers do not cause hyperglycaemia.

21 Features of Down's syndrome **Answers: A B C E**

Down's syndrome is due to trisomy of chromosome 21. It occurs in about 1 in 1000 live births; meiotic non-dysjunction is responsible for 90% of cases and is related to maternal age. There is a characteristic facies with a flat face, slanting eyes and epicanthic folds. There may be a single transverse palmar crease. A webbed neck occurs in Turner's syndrome (45 XO).

Down's syndrome is associated with congenital heart disease, which occurs in about 40% of cases. These include Tetralogy of Fallot (10%), patent ductus arteriosus (10%), ventricular septal defect (25%), atrial septal defect and endocardial cushion defects (40%).

The following are also features of, or occur more commonly in, Down's syndrome: acute lymphoblastic leukaemia, mental impairment, cataracts, epilepsy, scoliosis, duodenal atresia.

The anaesthetic implications mainly concern the airway. Intubation may be difficult due to a big tongue and small mouth. Atlanto-axial subluxation with instability occurs in about 15%. Sub-glottic stenosis may occur, necessitating an endotracheal tube of a smaller diameter than usual.

22 Medical complications of bronchial carcinoma include — Answers: A C D E

Carcinoma of the bronchus most commonly presents with haemoptysis and weight loss in a heavy smoker. The prognosis is poor, unless the tumour is localised and resectable. Most tumours respond poorly to either chemo- or radiotherapy, and many have metastasised to bone or other organs at the time of diagnosis. A patient with a Pancoast tumour in the apex of the lung invading the brachial plexus may present with Horner's syndrome.

There are many non-metastatic paraneoplastic syndromes that can occur in lung cancer including autonomic neuropathy, cerebellar degeneration, peripheral neuropathy and Eaton–Lambert syndrome. In about 10% of tumours there may be production of ectopic hormones such as ADH or parathormone. Clubbing and hypertrophic pulmonary osteoarthropathy can occur. Although not common, a lymphocytic meningitis can occur.

23 A fixed low cardiac output state — Answers: C E

A fixed low cardiac output state occurs in constrictive pericarditis and aortic stenosis. In anaemia there is a compensatory increase in cardiac output to maintain tissue oxygen delivery.

In Paget's disease there is often high output cardiac failure. The abnormal bone has such a huge vasculature that it puts great demands on the myocardium and the cardiac output is increased to such an extent as to cause the heart to fail.

Eisenmenger's syndrome occurs when pulmonary hypertension develops in the context of a long-standing ventricular septal defect. The result is a reversal of the shunt so that the shunt becomes right to left. This results in an elevated cardiac output.

24 A 'pink puffer', when compared with a 'blue bloater', will have — Answer: E

The classical 'pink puffer', when compared with the 'blue bloater', retains the drive to respiration that CO_2 produces on the central medullary respiratory centre. Thus the 'pink puffer' has a lower P_aCO_2 and a higher P_aO_2, compared to the 'blue bloater'.

Because the 'blue bloater' tends to be hypoxic, he or she has a higher haematocrit (secondary polycythaemia usually occurs). The hypoxia of the 'blue bloater' leads to pulmonary hypertension and cor pulmonale.

In reality the 'pink puffer' and 'blue bloater' represent two ends of a spectrum in chronic obstructive airways disease, and most patients have characteristics of both.

25 Peak flow **Answers: B C D E**

Peak flow is measured by the pneumotachograph. It is reduced in an acute attack of asthma and may be used to monitor the response to therapy. There is a diurnal variation in peak flow, caused by the diurnal variation in cortisol levels, which are lowest in early morning. This may cause morning dipping and episodes of wheezing in asthmatics. The measurement of peak flow is very operator dependent, and may be artefactually low in weak and debilitated patients.

26 Glycosuria **Answers: A B C D E**

Glycosuria occurs in diabetes mellitus and any cause of secondary diabetes such as acromegaly, phaeochromocytoma, Cushing's syndrome, steroid therapy, thiazides and haemochromatosis. Glycosuria occurs in pregnancy, following partial gastrectomy and pancreatectomy, and may occur following head injury as part of the body's general stress response.

27 Chronic renal failure **Answers: B C D E**

This topic was covered in answer 13. Chronic renal failure causes a normochromic, normocytic anaemia. Patients have hypergastrinaemia gastric erosions and may therefore have an iron deficiency anaemia. It may be secondary to or cause hypertension. It causes defective platelet function and a bleeding diathesis as a result. As a result of the metabolic acidosis of renal failure there is a right shift of the oxygen–haemoglobin dissociation curve. The hypocalcaemia of chronic renal failure induces secondary hyperparathyroidism.

28 Thrombolytic therapy — Answers: C E

Thrombolytic therapy is given to treat acute myocardial infarction. Streptokinase, tissue-type plasminogen activator (rt-PA) and APSAC (anistreplase) are the three commonly available thrombolytic agents. No one agent has been shown to be superior to the others.

Aspirin has an additive effect when combined with streptokinase in terms of reducing mortality. Thrombolytic therapy is contraindicated if there has been recent surgery, trauma or haemorrhage. Streptokinase cannot be given for a second time within 3 months of the previous dose, because of the risk of serious allergic reactions.

Malignant ventricular arrhythmias are very rare, but so-called reperfusion arrhythmias do occur following thrombolytic therapy.

29 Aortic regurgitation — Answer: E

In aortic regurgitation patients complain of dyspnoea, palpitations, chest pain (in the absence of coronary atheroma) and dizziness. Although the stroke volume is increased it is not a threefold increase. The murmur is an early blowing diastolic murmur, maximal on held expiration, sitting forward and in the 3rd or 4th intercostal space. There may be an associated diastolic thrill. The pressure gradient across the valve is in diastole, not systole.

30 Pulmonary fibrosis — Answers: A B C E

The causes of pulmonary fibrosis include the drugs busulphan, bleomycin, cyclophosphamide, nitrofurantoin, amiodarone, beryllium and paraquat, to name but a few. Steroids are sometimes used to treat pulmonary fibrosis. Pulmonary fibrosis is associated with autoimmune and connective tissue diseases and occupational dusts.

31 Platelet administration — Answers: A D

Platelets may be transfused to patients with acute thrombocytopenia, for instance in the context of postoperative bleeding. Platelets should be administered using a special filter. They do not require cross-matching, but must be group compatible. Platelets contain citrate as an anticoagulant.

Although platelets contain histamine, platelet administration does not result in any significant increase in plasma histamine. Platelets have a short shelf life, and need to be administered within a few days of collection.

32 Effective cardiopulmonary resuscitation — Answer: A

In effective mouth-to-mouth resuscitation, the percentage of inspired oxygen is about 14%. The expired CO_2 (ie the patient's) will be much greater than 2% because they are likely to have been apnoeic for some time.

The patient will have both a respiratory and metabolic acidosis: due to apnoea and anaerobic tissue metabolism, respectively. The pH of the blood will be less than 7.4, which is the normal plasma pH. The mixed venous oxygen saturation (S_vO_2) in a normal individual is about 75%. In a patient receiving effective mouth-to-mouth resuscitation the S_vO_2 would be unlikely to be greater than 75%. It is extremely unlikely that the systolic blood pressure will be anything approaching 100 mmHg.

33 Glutamine — Answers: B D

Glutamine is a non-essential amino acid, although in times of physiological stress it may become conditionally essential!

It constitutes 60% of free intracellular amino acids in skeletal muscle.

Glutamine is the principal metabolic fuel of gut mucosal cells (enterocytes), lymphocytes and monocytes. Recent studies have suggested that addition of glutamine to nutritional regimes may improve outcome in patients with sepsis and after surgery. It is possible that some of the immune dysfunction seen after trauma and sepsis is due to glutamine deficiency.

Coeliac disease is due to allergy to gluten.

Ref: O'Leary M J and Coakley J H. Nutrition and immunonutrition. *Br J Anaesth* 1996; **77**: 118–127.

34 Salicylate poisoning — Answers: A B E

Severe salicylate poisoning can cause profound metabolic upset. The acid–base status of the patient who has taken an aspirin overdose depends on the amount of drug taken. In mild overdose, the patient usually hyperventilates leading to a respiratory alkalosis, as the aspirin directly stimulates the respiratory centre in the brain. In severe aspirin overdose however, there is usually a metabolic acidosis due to uncoupling of oxidative phosphorylation. The blood gases may thus show a mixed respiratory alkalosis and metabolic acidosis.

Hypoprothrombinaemia occurs, for which intravenous vitamin K should be given, along with fresh frozen plasma. Thrombocytopenia may occur or there may be impaired platelet function. The serum fibrinogen is normal, and haemolysis does not occur. There may be gastrointestinal bleeding as a result of the coagulopathy.

35 Acute respiratory distress syndrome (ARDS) Answers: A C E

ARDS is characterised by refractory hypoxia (P_aO_2/F_iO_2 ratio <26.6 kPa), with bilateral diffuse pulmonary infiltrates on the CXR, a pulmonary artery wedge pressure of <18 mmHg (ie excluding heart failure or fluid overload as causes) in the context of a recognised risk factor for the development of the syndrome.

The lung compliance is markedly reduced. Thus in a patient with ARDS there is hypoxia, hypercarbia, reduced lung compliance, increased airway resistance and reduced diffusion capacity.

36 Anaphylaxis Answers: A E

The Association of Anaesthetists of Great Britain and Ireland revised guidelines on the management of suspected anaphylactic reactions associated with anaesthesia in 2003.

Initial therapy:

(a) stop administration of drug(s) likely to have caused the anaphylaxis
(b) maintain airway; give 100% oxygen
(c) lay patient flat with feet elevated
(d) give adrenaline
(e) start intravascular volume expansion with crystalloid or colloid.

Chlorpheniramine and hydrocortisone are second-line drugs.

37 Nitric oxide Answers: C E

Nitric oxide (NO) is a widespread biological mediator. It is synthesised from L-arginine by NO synthases, of which there are three types: endothelial (constitutive), neuronal and macrophage (inducible). NO is a highly reactive free radical with a half-life of a few seconds. NO was formerly known as endothelin-derived relaxant factor (EDRF). As the name implies it has a pivotal role in the maintenance of vascular tone in both the pulmonary and peripheral circulations. It inhibits platelet aggregation and is a vasodilator. NO stimulates guanylate cyclase leading to increased formation of cyclic GMP, which then acts at the cellular level to cause vasodilatation, as well as many other effects. NO is the final pathway for the action of glyceryl trinitrate and other nitrovasodilators. NO is one of the mediators in the sepsis syndrome causing peripheral vasodilatation. In very low concentrations (around 100 parts per billion) nitric oxide gas has been used to cause selective pulmonary vasodilatation and improve oxygenation. Paradoxically, perhaps, inhibitors of NO synthase such as L-NMMA (N^G-monomethyl L-arginine) have been used to correct the peripheral circulatory failure seen in sepsis syndrome.

NO is also a peripheral and central neurotransmitter at nitrergic neurones. It may play a part in the pathogenesis of such diverse conditions as diabetes mellitus, atherosclerosis, hypertension, Alzheimer's disease, Parkinson's disease and stroke.

Ref: Allen J D and Herity N A. Prospects for management of peripheral vascular failure in septic shock. *Br J Anaesth* 1996; **76**: 177–178.

38 Pulmonary artery occlusion pressure — Answer: D

The pulmonary artery occlusion pressure (PAOP) is measured with a flow-directed pulmonary artery catheter. Assuming that there is an uninterrupted column of blood from the pulmonary artery to the left atrium then the PAOP should be an accurate reflection of left atrial pressure (LAP). As long as there is no pressure gradient across the mitral valve then LAP should equal left ventricular end-diastolic pressure (LVEDP).

The final assumption in the measurement of PAOP is that, in the normally compliant left ventricle, a constant relationship (exponential not linear) holds between LVEDP and left ventricular end-diastolic volume.

Thus measurement of PAOP assumes that: PAOP=LAP=LVEDP≈LVEDV.

This does not always hold true. In myocardial infarction, cardiomyopathy and severe aortic regurgitation, the compliance of the left ventricle is reduced and LVEDP does not equate with LVEDV. In mitral stenosis the LAP is elevated and so PAOP/LAP does not reflect LVEDP.

39 Variables used in the APACHE III score include — Answers: C E

The prognosis for a group of patients admitted to ITU with a specific diagnosis is based on the APACHE III scoring system. APACHE stands for acute physiology and chronic health evaluation. In the original APACHE I there were 34 physiological variables. This was reduced to 12 in APACHE II. APACHE III included a further 6 variables. The 12 variables in APACHE II are: rectal temperature, mean arterial pressure, heart rate, respiratory rate, arterial pH, arterial P_aO_2, serum sodium, potassium and creatinine, haematocrit, white cell count and Glasgow coma scale. APACHE III adds urine output, whether the patient was intubated, serum urea, albumin, bilirubin and glucose, but does away with serum potassium.

40 Endotoxin **Answers: B D E**

Endotoxin is the part of a micro-organism which if present in sufficient amounts in the bloodstream will lead to the development of the sepsis syndrome, characterised by peripheral circulatory failure with systemic hypotension, pulmonary hypertension, pyrexia, tachycardia and either leucopenia or a neutrophil leucocytosis. Endotoxin is not invariably found in septic patients, but the test for its presence does use crab's blood!

The presence of endotoxin is thought to lead to the production of cytokines and other inflammatory mediators. In particular nitric oxide (NO) and the cytokines interleukin-6 (IL-6) and tumour necrosis factor-alpha (TNF) are thought to play an important part in the pathogenesis of the sepsis syndrome.

Although no longer available, an antibody directed against the A antigen of endotoxin was used as a treatment for sepsis. A trial looking at the efficacy of using this monoclonal antibody (called HA-1A, Centoxin) in patients with Gram-negative septicaemia was suspended.

41 Flail chest **Answers: C D**

In a patient with flail chest, being ventilated and losing 1.5 l/min, treatment might include increasing fresh gas flow by 1.5 l/min and reducing peak inspiratory flow rate.

42 Paracetamol poisoning **Answers: A B D E**

The most serious problem with paracetamol overdose is hepatotoxicity.

This is due to a toxic metabolite of paracetamol metabolism by the liver, which is normally scavenged by intracellular glutathione. In overdose the supply of glutathione is exhausted and the toxic metabolite then causes hepatocellular centrilobular necrosis. *N*-Acetylcysteine and methionine will act to mop up the toxic metabolite and prevent hepatic damage.

The hepatic damage, if it occurs, is not apparent until 48 h after the overdose. It causes a rise in the liver enzymes and a prolongation of the prothrombin time. The prothrombin time may be used to assess the degree of liver damage and may also be of prognostic value. In the most severe cases fulminant hepatic necrosis may occur, and liver transplant may be necessary.

43 Weaning from mechanical ventilation **Answers: C**

About 20% of all ventilated patients fail to be weaned initially. There are many reasons why such patients fail to wean. Impaired respiratory muscle strength may be due to malnutrition, acidosis, hypoxia or hypomagnesaemia, hypophosphataemia or hypocalcaemia. Factors such as bronchospasm or pulmonary oedema increase the load on the respiratory muscles and make successful weaning unlikely. The level of consciousness is important, and patients who are sedated are unlikely to wean rapidly. One bedside assessment of respiratory muscle strength is the P_{imax}. Most adults can achieve –100 cmH_2O. A severely weak patient might generate a P_{imax} of –20 cmH_2O. A P_{imax} of –30 cmH_2O suggests that a patient might wean.

44 The treatment of ARDS **Answers: A B C D E**

All these modalities have been tried – although none has been shown to provide enough benefit to be adopted universally. IVOX is intravenous oxygenation via a device placed in the vena cava. Kinetotherapy is the slow moving of the patient from side to side in the bed.

45 Concerning tetanus **Answers: C**

Tetanospasmin is the toxin responsible for the clinical manifestations of tetanus which results in rigidity due to inhibition of descending neurones within the spinal cord. More than 90% of patients admitted to ICU survive following which they will require immunisation as natural infection does not confer immunity.

46 The following support the diagnosis of fat embolism syndrome **Answers: B C D**

The petechial rash is characteristically over the head, trunk and arms. The ECG may show signs of right heart strain.

47 Concerning high-frequency jet ventilation (HFJV) **Answers: A B D E**

The expiratory phase is passive in contrast to high-frequency oscillation which employs higher frequency and active expiration and is used in neonates.

47 Concerning weakness associated with ICU care **Answers: A D**

Critical illness neuropathy is the commonest cause of weakness associated with ICU care and is commonly precipitated by SIRS. Creatinine phosphokinase is markedly raised in necrotising myopathy of ICU which is rare and may represent a very severe form of thick filament myopathy.

49 Causes of pulmonary hypertension include **Answers: B E**

It is mitral stenosis which causes pulmonary venous congestion and subsequent hypertension. A patent ductus arteriosus causes pulmonary hypertension due to increased pulmonary blood flow. Epoprostenol along with NO is used to treat pulmonary hypertension by causing pulmonary vasodilatation.

50 Concerning catheter-related blood stream infections (CR-BSI) **Answers: B E**

Staphylococci account for more than 50% of CR-BSI and catheters impregnated with chlorhexidine/silver or minocycline/rifampicin are effective in reducing infections though there are doubts relating to microbial resistance. Endoluminal brush sampling may generate a bacteraemia from a colonised line.

51 Trigeminal neuralgia **Answers: B C E**

Trigeminal neuralgia is an agonising pain in the distribution of the trigeminal (5th) cranial nerve, usually triggered from a place on the lips or the side of the nose. It is purely sensory, usually unilateral and does not affect the corneal reflex. It occurs mainly in the elderly; in a patient under 50 years old it may be symptomatic of multiple sclerosis. It may be relieved by carbamazepine or phenytoin. If medical therapy fails the patient may need phenol or glycerol injection into, section or radiofrequency ablation of, the trigeminal nerve. The pain may be so severe that the patient contemplates suicide.

52 Halothane **Answers: B C D E**

Halothane is a halogenated hydrocarbon. Its chemical formula is 2-bromo, 2-chloro, 1, 1, 1-trifluoroethane. It has a MAC of 0.76, a blood gas solubility coefficient of 2.4, a boiling point of 50°C, and a saturated vapour pressure of 32 kPa. It is unstable in light and therefore stored in dark bottles. It contains 0.01% thymol as a preservative. It is a bronchodilator and after sevoflurane is the least irritant to the respiratory tract of all the volatile agents. It inhibits hypoxic vasoconstriction, as do all the volatile agents.

It is a potent depressant of myocardial contractility. It may cause a nodal bradycardia, and in addition sensitises the myocardium to the action of catecholamines; arrhythmias are common. Halothane causes hypotension and inhibits the baroreceptor reflex, preventing a compensatory tachycardia. Halothane is 20% metabolised by the liver.

In up to 25% of patients exposed to halothane, there may be a mild, subclinical hepatitis, with jaundice and elevated liver enzymes. Rarely, a fulminating hepatic necrosis may occur which has a high mortality.

53 Pharmacokinetics of alfentanil and fentanyl **Answers: C D**

Alfentanil has a smaller volume of distribution (Vd) and a lower pK_a than fentanyl. It therefore has a faster onset, and a shorter duration of action. Alfentanil is less potent as it is less lipid soluble. Alfentanil is 92% protein bound, while fentanyl is 84% protein bound.

54 Plasma cholinesterases **Answers: A B C E**

Several anaesthetic agents are metabolised by plasma cholinesterases. Suxamethonium is the best known example, but all the ester local anaesthetics, including cocaine, are also metabolised this way.

Mivacurium, a non-depolarising muscle relaxant, and esmolol, a short-acting beta blocker, undergo metabolism by cholinesterases. So does aspirin!

Ref: Davis L, Britten J J and Morgan M. Cholinesterase. Its significance in anaesthetic practice. *Anaesthesia* 1997; **52**: 244–260.

55 Transdermal drugs **Answers: B D E**

Many drugs can be administered transdermally. Glyceryl trinitrate is often administered as small patches. Hyoscine patches are used as a treatment for motion sickness. Transdermal fentanyl patches are available for pain control in cancer patients.

56 The rhesus system — Answers: A B

The rhesus system describes the presence of (rhesus positive) or absence of (rhesus negative) the rhesus antigen on the surface of the red blood cells. The ABO system is the other major red cell antigen system used in transfusion medicine. A patient who is blood group O rhesus-negative does not have A, B or rhesus antigens on the surface of their blood cells.

They are thus the universal donor, as the lack of red antigens precludes any immunological response by a recipient. Because O rhesus-negative patients have no red cell antigens they therefore recognise A, B and rhesus as foreign and therefore have anti-A and anti-B antibodies (agglutinins) in their serum. Rhesus antibodies, however, only result from previous transfusion or pregnancy.

The Kell antigen is part of a lesser antigen system: the Kell, Kidd and Duffy system. There is no reason why an O rhesus-negative patient should have anti-Kell antibodies.

57 Sickle cell disease — Answer: A

A low haemoglobin in the absence of significant blood loss in an Afro-Caribbean male points to a possible diagnosis of sickle cell disease (SCD). The diagnosis is easily confirmed by a Sickledex test, which will, if positive, confirm the presence of sickle haemoglobin (Hb S). To quantify the amount of Hb S, haemoglobin electrophoresis is necessary.

Traditionally it has been taught that perioperative management should aim to avoid sickling conditions: hypoxia, acidaemia, hypothermia and dehydration, and has advocated (with very little clinical evidence) exchange transfusion, bicarbonate infusions and avoidance of tourniquets.

More recently the concept of the disease as one defined by chronic inflammatory vascular damage has emerged, calling into question the traditional dogma. Obviously hypoxia, acidaemia, hypothermia and dehydration should be avoided, but the necessity of exchange transfusions and avoidance of tourniquets has been seriously questioned, and bicarbonate is very unfashionable.

Transfusion to a preoperative Hb of 10 g/dl in a patient with a chronic Hb of 7.9 g/dl is unnecessary and potentially hazardous. Transfused blood is deficient in 2,3-DPG and so may impair tissue oxygenation.

Essential Ref: Firth P G. Anaesthesia for peculiar cells – a century of sickle cell disease. *Br J Anaesth* 2005; **95** (3): 287–299.

http://bja.oxfordjournals.org/cgi/reprint/95/3/287

58 Spinal anaesthesia — Answers: A B C D

Spinal anaesthesia results in loss of the vasoconstrictor tone in the circulation in the lower limbs, due to autonomic blockade. This may lead to hypotension, which can be counteracted by the administration of intravenous fluid (preloading), or by a vasoconstrictor such as ephedrine or methoxamine. If the spinal block is high enough to block the cardiac accelerator fibres (T1–T4) bradycardia occurs leading to hypotension which may be corrected by atropine or glycopyrrolate. In obstetric anaesthesia it is important to avoid aortocaval compression, which, in combination with a spinal, may lead to profound hypotension.

Ref: McCrae A F and Wildsmith J A. Prevention and treatment of hypotension during central neural block. *Br J Anaesth* 1993; **70**: 672–680.

59 A 3.5-kg baby — Answers: C D E

In a neonate, the tidal volume is 5–7 mls/kg, dead space is about 2–3 mls/kg and a respiratory rate of 40. Blood volume is 80–100 ml/kg (ie about 10% of body weight).

The haemoglobin concentration at birth is about 18 g/dl. This rises by about 1.2 g/dl in the first week. It then declines to around 10 g/dl at 3 months. By the first year it is about 12 g/dl and thereafter increases until adolescence.

60 Stellate ganglion block — Answer: C

A stellate ganglion block produces:

- (a) a Horner's syndrome, ptosis, enophthalmos, miosis
- (b) temperature increase in the ipsilateral arm and hand due to vasodilatation
- (c) flushing of the conjunctiva and skin
- (d) nasal stuffiness.

There is not sufficient sympathetic blockade to produce postural hypotension. The light reflex involves the optic nerve and the parasympathetic fibres of the oculomotor nerve and so is unaffected by a stellate ganglion block.

61 Postoperative hypertension **Answers: A C**

There are numerous possible causes of postoperative hypertension. The common causes include:

(a) pain, inadequate analgesia
(b) pre-existing hypertension, inadequately treated or as yet undiagnosed
(c) hypothermia, hypoxia or hypercarbia
(d) a full bladder.

Although phaeochromocytoma is a cause of postoperative hypertension it is extremely uncommon.

62 Action of drugs on the uterus **Answers: A C D**

The uterus consists of smooth muscle and therefore receives its motor innervation from the autonomic nervous system. There is no striated muscle and so neither suxamethonium nor any of the non-depolarising neuromuscular blocking drugs will have any effect on the uterus. The sympathetic outflow to the uterus comes from L2, L3 and L4. The uterus is also affected by the hormone oxytocin from the posterior pituitary. Oxytocin causes contraction of the uterus. The synthetic equivalent is generally used in obstetric anaesthetic practice. Syntocinon® also causes tachycardia and hypotension. Prostaglandins will cause contraction of the uterus.

The action of sympathetic nerves on the uterus is via beta-2 receptors.

Salbutamol and ritodrine both stimulate beta-2 receptors causing uterine relaxation. These agents can therefore be used to antagonise the effects of ergometrine. Isoflurane, like all the volatile agents, causes uterine relaxation.

63 Contraindications to suxamethonium **Answer: A**

The unwanted effects of suxamethonium include:

(a) myalgia postoperatively
(b) hyperkalaemia
(c) malignant hyperthermia

(d) anaphylaxis
(e) suxamethonium apnoea

In terms of contraindications, a patient known to have allergy to suxamethonium, and patients in whom hyperkalaemia would be especially dangerous should not receive the drug. There are a number of myopathic conditions in which suxamethonium is contraindicated.

Dystrophia myotonica is one such condition, as is myotonia congenita.

There is increased sensitivity to the drug in the Eaton–Lambert syndrome, and it should be avoided.

Suxamethonium does not precipitate porphyria, nor is it contraindicated in sickle cell disease, the neonate or in congestive cardiac failure.

64 Laparoscopic surgery **Answers: A B C D E**

Laparoscopic surgery leads to physiological changes as a result of insufflation of the abdomen with a gas, under pressure, often with the patient in the Trendelenburg position. Thus, the effects of the gas (usually CO_2) include gas embolism, hypercarbia and postoperative shoulder tip pain. The hypercarbia may predispose to arrhythmias and produce an acidosis. The fact that the gas is under pressure predisposes to pneumothorax or pneumomediastinum.

There is reduced thoracic compliance and the airway pressures are elevated. This increases the risk of barotrauma. It also leads to a reduction in functional residual capacity with shunting of blood and hypoxia. The pressure in the peritoneum may be sufficient to reduce venous return, cardiac output and blood pressure. More commonly however, if the patient is in the Trendelenburg position, there is a tachycardia with hypertension.

Intraperitoneal pressure should be monitored and should not exceed 30 cmH_2O. There is an increased risk of regurgitation if the patient is in the Trendelenburg position. Haemorrhage and perforation of a viscus can occur due to damage by the trocar.

65 Total hip replacement **Answers: A C**

Total hip replacement can be carried out under regional or general anaesthesia. There is no evidence that regional anaesthesia reduces long-term mortality. Although useful analgesics, NSAIDs may precipitate acute renal failure in the elderly or dehydrated patient. Hyperventilation is of no benefit and in the elderly may cause cerebral vasoconstriction with the risk of stroke. Methyl methacrylate cement may be used in total hip replacement. It is certainly not a positive inotrope.

Intra-operative embolism is not uncommon in this operation and will cause hypoxia. There is usually a tachycardia, hypotension and a sudden drop in end-tidal CO_2 when an embolus occurs.

66 Nerve damage in the lithotomy position — Answers: A D

The lithotomy position may result in nerve damage on the medial or the lateral side of the leg from pressure exerted by the stirrups. The common peroneal (lateral popliteal nerve) may be damaged in this position leading to foot drop, caused by compression of the nerve between the lithotomy pole and the head of the fibula. The saphenous nerve may be damaged if it is trapped between the lithotomy pole and the medial tibial condyle.

Ref: Warner M A, Martin J T, Schroeder D R, Offord K P and Chute C G. Lower-extremity motor neuropathy associated with surgery performed on patients in a lithotomy position. *Anesthesiology* 1994; **81**: 6–12.

67 Isoprenaline — Answer: D

Isoprenaline produces a tachycardia by stimulating beta-1 adrenergic receptors in the heart. Its action may thus be blocked by the beta-blocking drug propranolol.

Trimetaphan is a ganglion-blocking drug used to reduce blood pressure, which usually results in a compensatory tachycardia.

Atropine is vagolytic, used to treat bradycardia, and will thus exacerbate any tachycardia caused by isoprenaline.

Nifedipine is a calcium-channel-blocking drug used to reduce blood pressure. It usually produces a reflex tachycardia.

Phentolamine is an antagonist at alpha-1 adrenoreceptors, and when used to treat hypertension can cause a dramatic tachycardia.

68 Hepatitis B transmission — Answers: A B D E

The risk of transmission of hepatitis B has been reduced over the years by careful screening of all blood donors for hepatitis B sAg. Despite this there remains a small risk of viral transmission unless the blood products are pasteurised, heat treated, or treated by some other virucidal procedure.

Thus hepatitis B may be transmitted by platelets, packed red cells, plasma (FFP), fibrinogen and cryoprecipitate and human factor VIII. Factor VIII produced by recombinant DNA technology is totally free of risk as regards hepatitis B transmission.

69 The femoral nerve — Answers: A D

The femoral nerve is derived from the anterior primary rami of L2, L3 and L4, and is the largest nerve of the lumbar plexus. It enters the thigh beneath the inguinal ligament and lies 1 cm lateral to the femoral artery, outside the femoral sheath. A 3 in 1 block is a femoral nerve block with a large volume of local anaesthetic (20–30 ml) which diffuses within a single musculo-fascial plane to block the obturator and lateral cutaneous nerve of the thigh. Most of the foot is supplied by the sciatic nerve.

70 Side-effects of amiodarone — Answers: A B C D E

Amiodarone is a class III anti-arrhythmic in the Vaughan Williams classification of anti-arrhythmic agents. It is used to treat both ventricular and supraventricular arrhythmias. It has a number of side-effects; amongst the more benign are a photosensitive grey discoloration to the skin and reversible corneal micro-deposits. Amiodarone is an iodine-containing compound and it therefore can interfere with the thyroid gland. It can produce hypo- and hyperthyroidism. It can lead to potentially fatal pulmonary fibrosis, can cause hepatic dysfunction, and very rarely may cause a peripheral neuropathy.

71 Spinal block contraindications — Answers: A B C

None of the above are absolute contraindications to spinal block.

However, it is generally accepted that a spinal block can cause marked hypotension consequent upon the autonomic block that it produces. If there is existing hypovolaemia or the likelihood of significant blood loss (eg placenta praevia), a spinal block might lead to catastrophic hypotension, and thus it is a relative contraindication to its use in these instances. Although a regional technique is preferable to a general anaesthetic in pre-eclampsia, as it avoids the surge in blood pressure seen with laryngoscopy and intubation, an epidural is preferred to a spinal block as it is less likely to cause profound hypotension.

A breech presentation and fetal distress are not contraindications to a spinal block.

72 Tourniquets and nerve damage — Answers: C D E

Nerve damage from a tourniquet will produce signs of lower motor neurone damage. An extensor plantar response occurs in upper motor neurone damage. If there is nerve damage following the application of a tourniquet to the leg for 2 h the ankle jerk may be depressed.

There will be reduced pin prick at the toe and reduced vibration sense at the ankle. Stimulation of the common peroneal nerve will produce reduced movement at the ankle.

The Medical Defence Union makes the following recommendations:

(a) apply only to healthy limbs
(b) tourniquet size: arm 10 cm, leg 15 cm or wider in larger legs
(c) pressure: 50–100 mmHg above systolic for the arm; double systolic for the thigh OR arm 200–250 mmHg, leg 250–350 mmHg
(d) time: absolute maximum 3 h (recovers in 5–7 days); generally do not exceed 2 h
(e) documentation: duration and pressure at the least.

73 Hypertensive drug interaction with MAOIs — Answers: A D

Patients taking monoamine oxidase inhibitors as treatment for depression can develop severe hypertensive crises due to an interaction with ephedrine. The appropriate treatment for such a reaction includes using vasodilators to reverse the intense peripheral vasoconstriction responsible for the hypertension. Thus labetalol, phentolamine and diazoxide would all be of use in this situation.

74 Epidural analgesia — Answers: A B D

It is accepted that epidural analgesia may lead to both a prolonged second stage of labour and an increased rate of instrumental delivery.

What remains a disputed issue is whether there is an increased rate of caesarean section in parturients who receive epidural analgesia. The evidence to date suggests that there is no association between backache post-partum and the siting of an epidural. Both urinary retention and headache are potential complications of epidurals. The latter is due to inadvertent puncture of the dura and may require an epidural blood patch to treat it. There is a reduced rate of deep vein thrombosis with epidural anaesthesia.

Ref: McGrady E M. Extradural analgesia: does it affect progress and outcome in labour? *Br J Anaesth* 1997; **78**: 115–117.

Ref: *Fetal & Maternal Medicine Review* 1996; **8**: 29–55.

75 Adequacy of perfusion in posterior fossa surgery — Answers: B C E

If perfusion is reduced in posterior fossa surgery there is usually a rise in blood pressure (Cushing's reflex) in an attempt to compensate. There is often an associated bradycardia or arrhythmias and an abnormal respiratory pattern. Delta waves on the EEG are non-specific as the EEG is affected by so many other variables including the anaesthetic agents.

76 Propofol — Answers: A C D

Propofol is 2,6 di-isopropyl phenol. It is presented in a 1% solution (10 mg/ml) as a white emulsion containing soybean oil, egg phosphatide and glycerol. It is a rapidly acting intravenous anaesthetic agent with a rapid, clear recovery. It is metabolised mainly in the liver, but also in extrahepatic sites such as the lungs.

In terms of side-effects, it causes a 15%–25% drop in blood pressure by a reduction in cardiac output and systemic vascular resistance, which is of greater magnitude than that seen with thiopentone. It causes pain on injection and can cause green discoloration of the urine. It is not licensed for use in patients under the age of 3 years. It is safe in patients with malignant hyperpyrexia and in porphyria and patients with egg allergy, but should be avoided in patients with disorders of fat metabolism.

It has an anti-emetic action and in the CNS causes a reduction in cerebral blood flow, metabolism and intracranial pressure. It depresses laryngeal reflexes such that laryngeal mask insertion is facilitated and laryngospasm is uncommon.

77 Nitrous oxide — Answers: A C E

Nitrous oxide (N_2O) is a colourless gas which is stored in French blue cylinders as a liquid at a pressure of 5400 kPa (54 bar). Nitrous oxide interacts with vitamin B_{12}, stopping its ability to act as a coenzyme for methionine synthetase. This enzyme is essential for DNA synthesis. Exposure to nitrous oxide for 6 h or longer may result in megaloblastic anaemia. Nitrous oxide also interferes with folic acid metabolism.

Because nitrous oxide is 35 times more soluble in blood than nitrogen, it will diffuse into air-filled cavities, such as the middle ear, faster than the nitrogen diffuses out. Thus the pressure in the middle ear will increase and therefore in tympanoplasty nitrous oxide is a relative contraindication.

78 Obesity **Answers: B E**

Obesity is a metabolic disease in which adipose tissue comprises a greater proportion of body tissue than normal. Obesity predisposes to ischaemic heart disease, hypertension and diabetes mellitus. Hiatus hernia is more common, predisposing to regurgitation of acidic stomach contents and subsequent pneumonitis. In addition there is a greater incidence of difficult intubation in the obese. Chest wall and lung compliance is reduced. The functional residual capacity (FRC) is reduced and falls further with anaesthesia causing the closing volume to encroach on the FRC during normal tidal ventilation. This leads to increased *V/Q* mismatch and hypoxaemia due to the large intrapulmonary shunt. The incidence of thromboembolic problems such as deep vein thrombosis and pulmonary embolus is increased and so obese patients should be given prophylactic heparin prior to anything except minor surgery. Venous access and regional blocks may be technically difficult, as may finding an adequately sized blood pressure cuff.

Ref: Shenkman Z, Shir Y and Brodsky J B. Perioperative management of the obese patient. *Br J Anaesth* 1993; **70**: 349–359.

79 Brachial plexus blocks **Answers: A C E**

A supraclavicular brachial plexus block is more likely than an axillary block to produce side-effects. Supraclavicular blocks can be complicated by:

- (a) pneumothorax
- (b) intravascular injection
- (c) phrenic nerve block
- (d) Horner's syndrome

Apart from intravascular injection, the axillary approach to the brachial plexus is relatively free of complications. The supraclavicular approach, however, produces the most complete anaesthesia of the brachial plexus.

80 Autonomic nervous system **Answers: A B C D**

The autonomic nervous system consists of the sympathetic and parasympathetic systems. Acetylcholine is the neurotransmitter at all ganglia, at postganglionic parasympathetic nerves, and at the sympathetic nerves innervating the sweat glands.

Noradrenaline is the neurotransmitter at postganglionic sympathetic nerves. Whilst the action of acetylcholine is mainly terminated by metabolism, that of noradrenaline is mainly terminated by re-uptake into the nerve terminal.

The noradrenaline produced by sympathetic nerve endings acts on cell surface receptors of either alpha or beta type. Activation of beta receptors leads in turn to activation of the enzyme adenylate cyclase. Beta-2 receptors are found in the uterus and their stimulation results in relaxation of the uterus.

81 The following are appropriate analgesic doses for an 8-kg baby **Answers: A D**

Drug	Route	Dose	×8 kg
Paracetamol	PO	20 mg/kg QDS	160 mg
Diclofenac	PR	1 mg/kg TDS	8 mg
Ibuprofen	PO	5 mg/kg QDS	40 mg
Morphine	IV bolus	0.1 mg/kg PRN	0.8 mg
Codeine	IM	1–1.5 mg/kg QDS	8–12 mg

82 Gabapentin **Answers: C D E**

Gabapentin's name leads to some confusion. Gabapentin is a structural analogue of GABA, but it does not have any direct action at GABA receptors and it does not block GABA uptake or metabolism. Its exact mechanism of action remains unknown, but it has been shown to modulate glutamate receptors (NMDA/AMPA). Originally developed as an anticonvulsant it is now more widely used to treat neuropathic pain, and may have a place in the treatment of acute pain.

83 Definitions **Answers: A E**

Dysaesthesia is an unpleasant or abnormal sensation with or without a stimulus. Pain in an area that lacks sensation is anaesthesia dolorosa. Paraesthesia is an abnormal sensation perceived without an apparent stimulus. Pain in the distribution of a nerve or group of nerves is neuralgia. Hyperalgesia is an increased response to a normally noxious stimulus.

84 Carcinoid syndrome **Answers: A B D E**

Carcinoid tumours may secrete 5HT, bradykinin, substance P, histamine or prostaglandins. The presentation depends on which substance the tumour predominantly secretes, and where the tumour is. If the heart is involved it is invariably the right side as 5HT is deactivated by the lung. Hyperglycaemia may be a presenting feature. Hypoglycaemia is a side-effect of octreotide, a drug commonly used to control symptoms as it blocks gastroenteropancreatic peptide release. Traditionally inotropes are avoided as they can cause increased peptide release.

85 Congenital heart disease with right to left shunt **Answers: A D**

With right to left shunt the balance of pulmonary to systemic vascular resistance is critical. A reduction of systemic resistance increases the shunt. For this reason neuraxial blocks are avoided. Inhaled nitric oxide is sometimes used to attempt to reduce the pulmonary vascular resistance, and therefore reduce the shunt. Intravenous induction of anaesthesia is more rapid than usual, and inhalational induction slower because of the shunt.

86 Syringe labelling in critical care areas **Answers: A C D E**

Muscle relaxants have red labels, vasopressors have violet (pink) labels. All the labels have black lettering, except suxamethonium and adrenaline which have coloured lettering on a black background.

87 Consent for anaesthesia **Answers: A E**

The amount and the nature of information that should be disclosed to the patient should be determined by the question: 'What would this patient regard as relevant when coming to a decision about which of the available options to accept?' At the end of an explanation about a procedure, patients should be asked whether they have any questions; any such questions should be addressed fully and details recorded.

A separate formal written consent form signed by the patient is not required for anaesthetic procedures that are done to facilitate another treatment.

Ref: *Consent for anaesthesia*, revised edition 2006. Association of Anaesthetists of Great Britain and Ireland.

88 Day surgery — Answers: A C

The NHS plan target of 75% of elective surgery being performed as day cases means that this will form a high proportion of the work of most Departments of Anaesthesia. Fitness for a procedure should relate to the patient's health as found at pre-assessment and not limited by arbitrary limits such as ASA status or age. There is still insufficient evidence to recommend the use of routine prophylactic anti-emetics in day-surgery practice except in certain patient groups. These include those with a strong history of postoperative nausea and vomiting and those undergoing certain procedures, eg laparoscopic sterilisation, laparoscopic cholecystectomy and tonsillectomy.

Central neural blockade can be used for day-stay surgery, particularly if 23-h stay is considered in the definition. Effective audit is an essential component of good day stay anaesthesia.

Ref: *Day surgery*, revised edition 2005. The Association of Anaesthetists.

89 Management of anaesthesia for Jehovah's Witnesses — Answers: A D E

Although transfusion of blood is specifically forbidden by the religion no opinion should be attributed to a patient simply because they are a member of a religious or political group. All patients should be consulted individually to ascertain what treatments they will accept, and these discussions carefully documented. The religion does not specifically forbid, eg blood salvage, transplantation, epidural blood patch and blood products – individuals making their own choices about these.

Anaesthetists are not bound to treat Jehovah's Witnesses, except in an emergency, but if they do 'opt-out' then it is their responsibility to arrange for another anaesthetist who is happy to proceed.

90 The following drugs have anticonvulsant effects — Answers: A C E

Midazolam, a benzodiazepine, is an agonist at the GABA receptor. Gabapentin is used as an anticonvulsant, but confusingly does not seem to work at the GABA receptor. Magnesium is a specific anticonvulsant in eclampsia. Morphine has no anticonvulsant effects and flumazenil, a benzodiazepine antagonist, may promote fits in epileptics who are on long-term benzodiazepine treatment.

Practice Paper 1: Clinical Viva Answers

Viva 1

Examiner 1

Summarise this lady's case
This is an elderly lady with significant cardiovascular pathology who has refused local anaesthesia. In the past she has suffered a myocardial infarction and an embolus to the right arm.

Clinical examination reveals that she is in atrial fibrillation, with probable mixed mitral valve disease and a degree of left ventricular failure.

Current medications are digoxin (for her AF), Frumil® (for her LVF) and warfarin (previous embolism).

Tell me about her ECG
You should go systematically through her ECG telling the examiner about the rate, rhythm, axis and any abnormalities.

There are no P waves seen and the rhythm is irregularly irregular. She is in atrial fibrillation. In addition, there is left ventricular hypertrophy. The voltage of the R wave in V1 and that of S in V5 are greater than 35 mm, fulfilling the voltage criteria for LVH.

Describe the CXR
Again, the examiner will expect you to go through it systematically.

Describe the cardiac outline, the lung fields and any obvious pathology

This is an AP film that shows evidence of heart failure. The heart appears to be enlarged. There is prominence of the pulmonary vessels and diffuse interstitial shadowing extending out from both hila into the lung fields. Some septal lines are seen and there is thickening of the horizontal fissure on the right. There is lack of clarity of the intra-pulmonary vessels and frank alveolar oedema in the right zone.

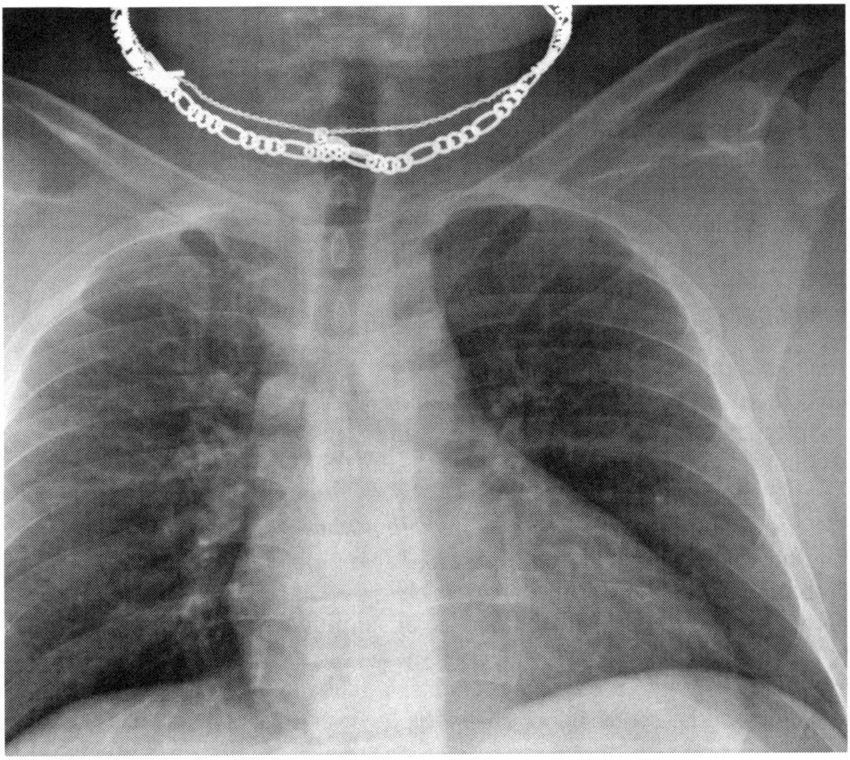

Fig. 3: Chest x-ray
Credit: Edward Kinsman/Science Photo Library

How would you anaesthetise this lady?
I would not anaesthetise this woman for an elective procedure today. She has a cardiac history, and some findings on examination and investigations of undiagnosed valvular heart disease and a degree of heart failure. Currently she poses a significant anaesthetic risk.

I propose that she have a cardiac echo and should be seen by a cardiologist with that result for optimisation of her AF, angina and heart failure medication, and for an opinion on the best management of her suspected valvular problems.

After full optimisation by the cardiologist the options for anaesthesia are either general or regional. She would need to have stopped her warfarin to be able to have a regional. Although this woman has previously refused a regional technique I would speak to her personally to establish her concerns.

Regional anaesthesia is generally considered safer in elderly patients having cataract surgery. She may find it more acceptable if she knew that I was present and could give some sedation.

If she still insists on a general anaesthetic the particular priorities are to minimise cardiac ischaemia by keeping pulse and blood pressure in the pre-operative range, and to avoid rises in intraocular pressure, by maintaining normocapnia – ventilating on an LMA if necessary, and avoiding compressing the neck veins.

Examiner 2

Tell me about premedication
This involves not only discussing anxiolytics (eg benzodiazepines) and analgesics (eg. Omnopon®) but also antisialagogues (eg hyoscine), anti-emetics (eg metoclopramide), EMLA cream, ranitidine, sodium citrate, etc.

Tell me about the anaesthetic complications following thyroidectomy
You need to discuss intra- and postoperative problems. The major group of problems includes airway problems, such as tracheal collapse, laryngeal nerve palsy causing stridor, and haematomas causing airway compression. You need to discus the management of each of these problems. Haematoma needs to be evacuated urgently. Stridor may require re-intubation which should be done as a controlled gaseous induction technique by an experienced anaesthetist.

How would you anaesthetise a 25-year-old asthmatic who has a blood pressure of 170/100 mmHg and is due to have an inguinal hernia repair?
The answer in simple terms is to defer the operation until the hypertension is controlled.

Viva 2: Model Answers

Examiner 1

Tell me about the anaemia of chronic renal failure
In chronic renal failure, there is usually a normochromic, normocytic anaemia. This is due to reduced production of erythropoietin (EPO) by the kidneys. As a compensatory mechanism to ensure adequate tissue oxygenation the oxyhaemoglobin dissociation curve shifts to the right.

This is facilitated by the metabolic acidosis that occurs and an increase in 2,3-DPG. The anaemia may be corrected by subcutaneous EPO produced by recombinant DNA technology, or by transfusion of red blood cells.

Tell me about the causes of delayed gastric emptying
Factors that may delay gastric emptying include:

Physiological factors
- Food
- Obesity
- Posture
- Pregnancy and labour

Pathological factors
- Anxiety
- Pain
- Shock
- Trauma
- Diabetic autonomic neuropathy
- Myxoedema
- Scleroderma
- Pyloric stenosis
- Electrolyte disturbance

Pharmacological factors
- Opioids
- Anticholinergic drugs
- Alcohol
- Tricyclic antidepressants
- Aluminium hydroxide

Examiner 2

Tell me about the anatomy of the caudal canal
The caudal space is a continuation of the epidural space. In the adult the spinal cord ends at L 1/2. The dural sac terminates at the level of the second sacral vertebra. Below this is the caudal space.

Failure of fusion of the laminae of the fifth sacral vertebra produces the sacral hiatus; a horseshoe-shaped indentation bounded laterally by the sacral cornua. Access to the space is via the sacrococcygeal membrane.

The caudal space contains veins, fat and the sacral nerve roots including S2, S3 and S4, which carry parasympathetic fibres and innervate the uterus and bladder.

Tell me about the problems of hypotensive anaesthesia
Hypotensive anaesthesia is employed to reduce blood loss and to facilitate visualisation of the surgical field in ENT, orthopaedic and microsurgical operations.

Contraindications include hypertension, ischaemic or valvular heart disease or a previous stroke. Hypovolaemia, pregnancy, anaemia, renal and hepatic disease are relative contraindications.

The problems encountered with hypotensive anaesthesia are due to reduced perfusion of vital organs if the blood pressure falls below the usual autoregulatory threshold.

The cerebral circulation autoregulates blood flow between a mean arterial blood pressure of 50 and 150 mmHg. Cerebral infarction (stroke) may occur in severe hypotension.

Coronary perfusion depends on many factors but in particular requires an adequate diastolic blood pressure. Hypotensive anaesthesia may thus precipitate myocardial ischaemia or infarction.

Renal perfusion ceases below a mean arterial blood pressure of 60 mmHg.

Short Answer Question Paper 2

1 How would you preoperatively assess (40%), investigate (20%) and resuscitate (40%) a 6-week-old infant prior to repair of congenital hypertrophic pyloric stenosis?

2 What are the preconditions and exclusions for brain stem death testing? (50%) How would you perform brain stem death testing? (50%)

3 A primigravid woman is found collapsed in the delivery suite following an epidural 'top-up' administered by the midwife 5 min before. List the likely causes (40%) and the initial management. (60%)

4 A previously fit 30-year-old male sustains an isolated fracture of the femur during a motorcycle accident. Six hours after admission he becomes dyspnoeic. What are the likely causes and their initial management?

5 Describe your management of an adult patient brought into the accident and emergency department in status epilepticus.

6 How may nutrition be provided for patients on the intensive care unit? (30%) What are the advantages and disadvantages of each? (70%)

7 What are the indications for awake intubation in the adult? (30%) How may the airway be anaesthetised prior to intubation? (70%)

8 How may gas exchange and anaesthesia be maintained during rigid bronchoscopy? (70%) What problems are associated with each method? (30%)

9 **How would you diagnose, treat and investigate a suspected case of suxamethonium apnoea?**

10 **Write brief notes on the complications of blood transfusion.**

11 **What are the options for postoperative analgesia following an open nephrectomy? (40%) State briefly the advantages and disadvantages of each. (60%)**

12 **What are the specific difficulties of anaesthetising an acromegalic patient for a transsphenoidal hypophysectomy?**

Multiple Choice Question Paper 2

1 The Severinghaus electrode

- ❑ A consists of CO_2-sensitive glass
- ❑ B is better with gases than blood
- ❑ C is affected by nitrous oxide
- ❑ D contains bicarbonate ions in the electrolyte solution
- ❑ E measures pH

2 Monitoring of evoked potentials

- ❑ A the stimulus can be auditory
- ❑ B the stimulus can be visual
- ❑ C the stimulus can be somatosensory
- ❑ D evoked potential signals have an amplitude of 10–300 μV
- ❑ E the signal is only revealed after summation of multiple repetitions

3 Helium

- ❑ A has similar viscosity to oxygen
- ❑ B causes changes in voice
- ❑ C is useful treatment for bronchospasm
- ❑ D is stored as a liquid
- ❑ E supports combustion

4 In an exponential process

- ❑ A time constant and half-life are synonymous
- ❑ B 37% of the process is completed in one time constant
- ❑ C 95% of the process is completed in three time constants
- ❑ D rate of change is constant
- ❑ E washout curves are exponential processes

5 The hazard of microshock in hospital can be reduced by the use of

- ❑ A isolated (floating) power supply
- ❑ B saline-filled intracardiac catheters
- ❑ C battery-powered appliances
- ❑ D multiple earth paths
- ❑ E large area diathermy plate

6 Mechanics

- ❑ A mass is a scalar quantity
- ❑ B weight is a vector quantity
- ❑ C acceleration is a scalar quantity
- ❑ D force is a vector
- ❑ E if the velocity of an object doubles, its kinetic energy also doubles

7 Surgical lasers

- ❑ A the effect on the tissues depends upon the laser light wavelength
- ❑ B CO_2 lasers can be directed through fibreoptic cables
- ❑ C argon laser light is readily absorbed by the cornea
- ❑ D Nd-YAG laser light has a wavelength of 1060 nm
- ❑ E when used in the airway the F_iO_2 should be kept as low as possible

8 Concerning the response of measurement systems

- ❑ A drift is defined as an error that is dependent on whether the measured value is increasing or decreasing
- ❑ B overdamping can result in oscillation and overestimation of the reading
- ❑ C critical damping is defined as the fastest response without overshoot
- ❑ D ideally the signal-to-noise ratio should be low
- ❑ E averaging over multiple samples may help to eliminate noise

9 Concerning intra-arterial blood pressure measurement

- ☐ A the transducer is a piezoresistive strain gauge type
- ☐ B the system is designed with a frequency response range of 40–200 Hz
- ☐ C air bubbles in the tubing increase the damping
- ☐ D arterial cannulae are designed to be compliant
- ☐ E false aneurysm is a late complication of arterial cannulation

10 In a positive (or upward or right) skewed distribution (such as might be found by asking a primary school class 'how many children live in your house?')

- ☐ A the median is greater than the mean
- ☐ B the mode is less than the mean
- ☐ C the mean is the best descriptor of central tendency
- ☐ D a logarithmic transformation may normalise the data
- ☐ E a square transformation may normalise the data

11 Carcinoid syndrome may be treated with

- ☐ A hydrocortisone
- ☐ B ketanserin
- ☐ C octreotide
- ☐ D Trasylol®
- ☐ E aspirin

12 Nimodipine

- ☐ A is a calcium antagonist
- ☐ B increases cerebral vasospasm
- ☐ C causes a reduced systemic vascular resistance
- ☐ D concomitant use of intravenous beta-blockers should be avoided
- ☐ E interferes with aminophylline

13 Constrictive pericarditis is associated with

- ☐ A pulsus paradoxus
- ☐ B tuberculosis
- ☐ C decreased myocardial contractility
- ☐ D pulmonary oedema
- ☐ E an elevated central venous pressure

14 Aortic regurgitation may occur in

- ❑ A Marfan's syndrome
- ❑ B rheumatoid arthritis
- ❑ C ankylosing spondylitis
- ❑ D syphilis
- ❑ E bacterial endocarditis

15 The incidence of deep vein thrombosis (DVT) is increased by

- ❑ A the oral contraceptive pill
- ❑ B HbSC disease
- ❑ C the lupus anticoagulant
- ❑ D polycythaemia
- ❑ E malignancy

16 Recognised features of acromegaly include

- ❑ A hypertension
- ❑ B glucose intolerance
- ❑ C dry skin
- ❑ D thyroid goitre
- ❑ E galactorrhoea

17 Diabetic autonomic neuropathy may result in

- ❑ A silent ischaemia
- ❑ B asystole
- ❑ C impotence
- ❑ D no pressor response to intubation
- ❑ E prolongation of the QT interval on the ECG

18 The bleeding time may be prolonged in

- ❑ A haemophilia A
- ❑ B von Willebrand's disease
- ❑ C disseminated intravascular coagulation (DIC)
- ❑ D vitamin K deficiency
- ❑ E scurvy

19 The following are found in primary hyperparathyroidism

- ❑ A extraosseous calcification
- ❑ B renal calculi
- ❑ C raised plasma calcium
- ❑ D lowered urinary calcium
- ❑ E increased urinary phosphate

20 Papilloedema can

- ❑ A be caused by central retinal artery occlusion
- ❑ B be caused by central retinal vein occlusion
- ❑ C be caused by cavernous sinus thrombosis
- ❑ D be unilateral
- ❑ E occur with pulmonary oedema

21 Blood cell antigen A

- ❑ A has Mendelian inheritance
- ❑ B is less common than B
- ❑ C is the main cause of haemolytic disease of the newborn
- ❑ D is found in all RBCs
- ❑ E is found in saliva

22 The following values are less in obstructive than in restrictive lung disease

- ❑ A functional residual capacity (FRC)
- ❑ B FEV_1/FVC
- ❑ C peak expiratory flow rate (PEFR)
- ❑ D carbon monoxide transfer factor (TLCO)
- ❑ E tidal volume (TV)

23 Erythropoietin production

- ❑ A is reduced in renal disease
- ❑ B is stimulated by hypercarbia
- ❑ C is increased in chronic obstructive airways disease
- ❑ D is reduced at altitude
- ❑ E takes place in the bone marrow

24 The following are associated with rheumatoid arthritis

- ❑ A pericardial effusion
- ❑ B haemolytic anaemia
- ❑ C constrictive pericarditis
- ❑ D renal failure
- ❑ E tricuspid incompetence

25 Concerning phaeochromocytoma

- ❑ A 10% are familial
- ❑ B they may cause hypotension
- ❑ C they may cause hypertension
- ❑ D they may secrete adrenaline, noradrenaline or dopamine
- ❑ E they are a cause of secondary diabetes insipidus

26 An increased tidal volume is usual in

- ❑ A ankylosing spondylitis
- ❑ B diabetic ketoacidosis
- ❑ C emphysema
- ❑ D cerebral haemorrhage
- ❑ E uraemia

27 Diabetic amyotrophy

- ❑ A affects predominantly the distal muscles of the lower limbs
- ❑ B is associated with an increase in cerebrospinal fluid protein
- ❑ C usually responds to improved blood sugar control
- ❑ D causes impotence
- ❑ E causes urinary retention

28 A patient who has vomited presents with acute abdominal pain. On examination he is noted to have epigastric guarding, laboured respiration, slight cyanosis and subcutaneous emphysema in the neck. This suggests

- ❑ A pulmonary infarction
- ❑ B ruptured diaphragm
- ❑ C spontaneous pneumothorax
- ❑ D ruptured oesophagus
- ❑ E ruptured trachea

29 Dystrophia myotonica is associated with

- ❑ A sterility
- ❑ B dysarthria
- ❑ C cataracts
- ❑ D temporalis muscle wasting
- ❑ E sternocleidomastoid muscle wasting

30 The following clinical findings occur in hemisection of the spinal cord (Brown-Sequard syndrome)

- ❑ A contralateral weakness
- ❑ B ipsilateral extensor plantar responses
- ❑ C contralateral loss of pain and temperature sensation
- ❑ D ipsilateral loss of awareness of vibration
- ❑ E Rombergism

31 The following blood gases values could be seen with aspirin poisoning

- ❑ A pH 6.9
- ❑ B P_aCO_2 3.2 kPa
- ❑ C P_aO_2 10 kPa
- ❑ D actual bicarbonate of 10 mmol/l
- ❑ E readings consistent with a base excess of +5

32 Measurement of cardiac output using a pulmonary artery catheter is affected by

- ❑ A the temperature of the patient
- ❑ B the temperature of the injectate
- ❑ C position of the proximal port
- ❑ D constrictive pericarditis
- ❑ E the skill of the operator

33 The following are appropriate treatment regimens

- ❑ A methionine for paraquat poisoning
- ❑ B assisted ventilation for salicylate poisoning
- ❑ C physostigmine for imipramine overdose
- ❑ D dicobalt edetate for cyanide poisoning
- ❑ E atropine for paracetamol poisoning

34 An elderly lady is dehydrated from prolonged intestinal obstruction. She is tachypnoeic and distressed, breathing air. The following are likely:

- ❑ A respiratory alkalosis
- ❑ B metabolic acidosis
- ❑ C hypoxaemia
- ❑ D uraemia
- ❑ E hyperglycaemia

35 Hypotension and an elevated central venous pressure may occur in

- ❑ A pulmonary embolism
- ❑ B haemorrhage
- ❑ C congestive cardiac failure
- ❑ D tension pneumothorax
- ❑ E myocardial infarction

36 In the management of adult VF arrest

- ❑ A the first shock should be 100 J
- ❑ B the first drug should be adrenaline 1 mg IV
- ❑ C early IV bicarbonate is recommended
- ❑ D bretylium tosylate is given in a dose of 5 mg/kg
- ❑ E isoprenaline is used in a dose of 5 μg/kg

37 In a patient with an acute spinal cord injury

- ❑ A suxamethonium is contraindicated
- ❑ B steroids improve prognosis
- ❑ C there is usually a tachycardia
- ❑ D more than 75% of patients develop autonomic hyperreflexia
- ❑ E hypotensive anaesthesia is desirable as it reduces blood loss

38 Myxoedema coma is treated with

- ❑ A intravenous thyroxine
- ❑ B oral thyroxine
- ❑ C intravenous saline
- ❑ D intravenous hydrocortisone
- ❑ E warming the patient

39 Fat embolism can cause

- ❑ A a petechial rash
- ❑ B central cyanosis
- ❑ C pyrexia
- ❑ D cerebral oedema
- ❑ E carbon dioxide retention

40 The following may cause convulsions

- ❑ A hypomagnesaemia
- ❑ B hypercalcaemia
- ❑ C ketamine
- ❑ D hyponatraemia
- ❑ E anaemia

41 The following would alert you to the need to increase respiratory support

- ❑ A tired and sweating
- ❑ B mouth open and tracheal tug
- ❑ C use of platysma
- ❑ D flaring of the ala nasae
- ❑ E bounding peripheral pulses

42 The following are essential criteria for brain stem death

- ❑ A equal pupils
- ❑ B absent limb movements
- ❑ C doll's eye movements
- ❑ D P_aCO_2 >6.7 kPa at the end of apnoea
- ❑ E normal blood glucose

43 The following may cause a metabolic alkalosis

- ❑ A Cushing's syndrome
- ❑ B gastrocolic fistula
- ❑ C acetazolamide
- ❑ D pyloric stenosis
- ❑ E carbenoxolone therapy

44 Disseminated intravascular coagulation (DIC) may occur in

- ❑ A amniotic fluid embolus
- ❑ B acute promyelocytic leukaemia
- ❑ C falciparum malaria
- ❑ D haemolytic transfusion reaction
- ❑ E thrombotic thrombocytopenic purpura

45 In acute liver failure

- ❑ A a prothrombin time >20 s indicates severe failure
- ❑ B the level of serum alanine aminotransferase (ALT) is a sensitive marker
- ❑ C the serum bilirubin is a sensitive marker
- ❑ D paracetamol may be implicated aetiologically
- ❑ E halothane may be implicated aetiologically

46 The following may be early complications of tracheostomy

- ❑ A pneumothorax
- ❑ B tracheal stenosis
- ❑ C haemorrhage
- ❑ D surgical emphysema
- ❑ E cardiovascular collapse

47 Left ventricular failure is a more likely diagnosis than asthma in the presence of

- ❑ A early cyanosis
- ❑ B a raised jugular venous pressure (JVP)
- ❑ C expiratory rhonchi
- ❑ D inspiratory basal crepitations
- ❑ E shadowing on the chest X-ray (CXR)

48 Concerning the oxyhaemoglobin dissociation curve

- ❑ A the P_{75} is 5.3 kPa
- ❑ B it is shifted to the right in chronic anaemia
- ❑ C it is shifted to the left in hypoventilation
- ❑ D it is unaffected by temperature
- ❑ E it is shifted to the right in carbon monoxide poisoning

49 Hypofibrinogenaemia occurs with

❑ A DIC
❑ B the oral contraceptive pill
❑ C asparaginase
❑ D prostate resection
❑ E massive transfusion

50 Two days post abdominal surgery the following observations are recorded: blood pressure 80/40 mmHg, pulse 100 beats/min, temperature 39°C, central venous pressure 2 cmH_2O. This could be due to

❑ A myocardial infarct
❑ B septicaemia
❑ C pneumonia
❑ D anastomotic breakdown
❑ E cardiac tamponade

51 The penicillins

❑ A are bacteriostatic
❑ B inhibit bacterial cell wall synthesis
❑ C are active only against Gram +ve organisms
❑ D rarely cause allergic reactions
❑ E are the treatment of choice for a UTI

52 The following are effective blocks for relieving the pain of chronic pancreatitis

❑ A coeliac plexus
❑ B lumbar sympathetic
❑ C thoracic epidural
❑ D paravertebral
❑ E stellate ganglion

53 Soda lime

❑ A contains 70% calcium hydroxide and 30% sodium hydroxide
❑ B may not be used with sevoflurane
❑ C produces humidification of inspired gases
❑ D may warm up to 60°C during active CO_2 absorption
❑ E use has been associated with carboxyhaemoglobinaemia

54 Sevoflurane

- ❑ A is an isomer of isoflurane
- ❑ B may cause nephrotoxicity due to its metabolism to fluoride ions
- ❑ C requires a heated vaporiser for its administration
- ❑ D is less potent than desflurane
- ❑ E causes tachycardia and hypertension at >1 minimum alveolar concentration

55 The following occur postoperatively

- ❑ A increase in nitrogen excretion
- ❑ B increase in K^+ excretion
- ❑ C increase in urinary sodium excretion
- ❑ D hyperglycaemia
- ❑ E sleep disturbances

56 The following suggest a difficult intubation

- ❑ A Mallampati grade 3
- ❑ B a thyromental distance of <6 cm
- ❑ C Wilson score >2
- ❑ D obesity
- ❑ E Parkinson's disease

57 Massive blood transfusion may cause

- ❑ A a coagulopathy
- ❑ B pulmonary damage
- ❑ C hypercalcaemia
- ❑ D alkalosis
- ❑ E renal failure

58 Acetylcholine is the neurotransmitter at

- ❑ A postganglionic sympathetic nerve fibres at the adrenal medulla
- ❑ B postganglionic sympathetic nerve fibres supplying sweat glands
- ❑ C postganglionic sympathetic nerve fibres supplying the bronchi
- ❑ D all autonomic ganglia
- ❑ E the neuromuscular junction

59 The following can be used to test the integrity of the autonomic nervous system

- ❑ A Valsalva manoeuvre
- ❑ B ephedrine
- ❑ C palpating a pulse
- ❑ D echocardiography
- ❑ E phentolamine

60 An adult patient with a prosthetic heart valve requires general anaesthesia for extraction of wisdom teeth. He should receive the following antibiotic cover

- ❑ A gentamicin only
- ❑ B amoxicillin and gentamicin
- ❑ C vancomycin and gentamicin, if allergic to penicillin
- ❑ D no antibiotic cover
- ❑ E teicoplanin alone

61 The following drugs are teratogens

- ❑ A lithium
- ❑ B warfarin
- ❑ C isoflurane
- ❑ D tetracyclines
- ❑ E carbamazepine

62 The following may be features of the TUR syndrome

- ❑ A hypotension with bradycardia
- ❑ B confusion
- ❑ C hypernatraemia
- ❑ D haemolysis
- ❑ E disseminated intravascular coagulation

63 Ropivacaine

- ❑ A has an identical p*K*a to bupivacaine
- ❑ B is less cardiotoxic than bupivacaine
- ❑ C is more potent than bupivacaine
- ❑ D produces greater motor block than bupivacaine
- ❑ E is a pure enantiomer

64 The recurrent laryngeal nerve

- ❑ A supplies the sensory fibres to the larynx below the vocal cords
- ❑ B supplies the motor fibres to some intrinsic muscles of the larynx
- ❑ C crosses the inferior thyroid artery or its branches
- ❑ D supplies the motor fibres to the cricothyroid muscle
- ❑ E supplies the inferior constrictor muscle of the pharynx

65 Lower oesophageal tone is increased by

- ❑ A metoclopramide
- ❑ B atropine
- ❑ C domperidone
- ❑ D morphine
- ❑ E cisapride

66 Magnesium

- ❑ A is the anticonvulsant of choice in eclampsia
- ❑ B readily crosses the placenta
- ❑ C potentiates the action of non-depolarising muscle relaxants
- ❑ D overdosage causes cardiac arrest
- ❑ E deficiency causes prolongation of the QT interval on the ECG

67 Radial nerve palsy causes

- ❑ A inability to extend the elbow
- ❑ B inability to extend the wrist
- ❑ C inability to pronate the forearm
- ❑ D loss of sensation at the base of the thumb
- ❑ E wasting of the thenar eminence

68 Non-steroidal anti-inflammatory drugs

- ❑ A are useful postoperative analgesics
- ❑ B may cause thrombocytopenia
- ❑ C can be given intrathecally
- ❑ D inhibit cyclooxygenase
- ❑ E can precipitate renal failure

69 Trigeminal neuralgia

❑ A affects the sixth cranial nerve
❑ B when the ophthalmic branch of the trigeminal nerve is affected there is loss of the corneal reflex
❑ C is successfully treated with carbamazepine
❑ D may be intractable
❑ E may be the presenting feature in multiple sclerosis

70 Etomidate

❑ A is an imidazole
❑ B has an ester link
❑ C causes greater postoperative nausea and vomiting than propofol
❑ D has a low incidence of allergy
❑ E is contraindicated in porphyria

71 Regarding malignant hyperpyrexia

❑ A it may be precipitated by nitrous oxide
❑ B it may be precipitated by isoflurane
❑ C dantrolene is the specific treatment
❑ D it is inherited as an autosomal recessive gene
❑ E the local anaesthetic agents are safe

72 Treatment of air embolism during posterior cranial fossa surgery includes

❑ A increasing intracranial venous pressure
❑ B rapid intravenous fluids
❑ C mannitol
❑ D placing the patient laterally, right side down
❑ E increasing the nitrous oxide

73 Amniotic fluid embolism

❑ A can occur more than 24 h after delivery
❑ B can occur after a therapeutic abortion
❑ C can only be diagnosed definitely at post mortem
❑ D is commoner if a Syntocinon® infusion is used
❑ E there is often an associated coagulopathy

74 Crystalloid cardioplegic solutions

- ❑ A contain high concentrations of calcium
- ❑ B contain high concentrations of potassium
- ❑ C contain procaine
- ❑ D stop the heart in diastole
- ❑ E may contain magnesium

75 Concerning an ankle block

- ❑ A there are four nerves to be blocked
- ❑ B apart from the saphenous nerve, all the other nerves to be blocked are derived from the sciatic nerve
- ❑ C the sural nerve lies anterior to the lateral malleolus
- ❑ D the tibial nerve lies deep to the posterior tibial artery
- ❑ E the deep peroneal nerve lies lateral to the anterior tibial artery

76 Concerning the neonatal airway

- ❑ A the trachea is 4 cm long
- ❑ B the larynx is at C5
- ❑ C the epiglottis is U-shaped
- ❑ D the tracheal rings are not fully formed
- ❑ E the cricoid is the narrowest part of the airway

77 Fallot's tetralogy is associated with

- ❑ A squatting
- ❑ B syncope
- ❑ C murmur due to continuous flow through a VSD
- ❑ D overriding pulmonary artery
- ❑ E aortic stenosis

78 Morphine

- ❑ A may cause inappropriate ADH release
- ❑ B is metabolised to morphine 6-glucuronide
- ❑ C is an antiemetic
- ❑ D stimulates the Edinger–Westphal nucleus
- ❑ E stimulates the chemoreceptor trigger zone

79 Retrobulbar block

- ❑ A prevents lacrimation
- ❑ B causes papilloedema
- ❑ C causes enophthalmos
- ❑ D decreases intraocular pressure
- ❑ E causes miosis

80 Myasthenia gravis

- ❑ A only occurs in females
- ❑ B is associated with anti-acetylcholine receptor antibodies
- ❑ C patients are resistant to non-depolarising muscle relaxants
- ❑ D may be treated by plasmapheresis
- ❑ E is often due to an underlying oat cell carcinoma of the bronchus

81 The following are standard IV induction doses for a 15-kg child

- ❑ A thiopentone 75 mg
- ❑ B atracurium 7.5 mg
- ❑ C suxamethonium 50 mg
- ❑ D fentanyl 15 mg
- ❑ E ketamine 30 mg

82 Foreign body inhalation

- ❑ A is most common in children
- ❑ B objects preferentially go to the right main bronchus
- ❑ C chest X-ray may show unilateral lung collapse
- ❑ D chest X-ray may show unilateral lung over inflation
- ❑ E removal is usually by flexible bronchoscopy

83 Anaesthesia for patients who have transplanted hearts

- ❑ A at rest a denervated heart usually beats faster than an innervated one
- ❑ B atropine is avoided as it causes exaggerated tachycardia
- ❑ C isoprenaline is a better choice than ephedrine to raise the heart rate
- ❑ D asepsis is even more important than usual
- ❑ E angina is rare in transplanted hearts

84 Management of severe pre-eclampsia

- ❑ A hypertension may be controlled with ramipril
- ❑ B treatment of hypertension does not halt the progress of the disease
- ❑ C if the platelet count is above 100×10^9/l without transfusion, the INR is usually normal
- ❑ D magnesium suppresses EEG excitatory activity
- ❑ E it has been shown that fluid resuscitation with colloid is superior to crystalloid

85 Cricoid pressure

- ❑ A the cricoid cartilage is at the level of C4
- ❑ B the cricoid cartilage forms the only complete ring in the larynx and trachea
- ❑ C the force required to prevent passive regurgitation is about 40 N
- ❑ D the force should be increased if there is active vomiting
- ❑ E it may make intubation easier

86 Association of Anaesthetists checklist for anaesthetic equipment (2004)

- ❑ A the first thing is to 'tug test' each gas pipeline
- ❑ B the breathing system must be checked before each new patient
- ❑ C the vaporiser must be checked before each new patient
- ❑ D the suction apparatus must be checked before each new patient
- ❑ E relevant checks should be recorded on each patient's anaesthetic chart

87 Platelet transfusion

- ❑ A is indicated in a patient requiring urgent surgery if the count is $<50 \times 10^9$/l
- ❑ B is indicated in an otherwise stable ITU patient if the count is $<50 \times 10^9$/l
- ❑ C is indicated to enable epidural analgesia to complement general anaesthesia
- ❑ D the risk of transfusion-related bacterial infection is higher than for other blood products
- ❑ E a 'pool' of platelets is the pooled buffy coats of the whole blood from 16 donors

88 Catastrophes in anaesthetic practice

- ❑ A most anaesthetists never experience the death of a patient 'on the table'
- ❑ B breaking bad news to relatives should be done immediately by telephone
- ❑ C a consultant unconnected with the case should check all drugs and equipment
- ❑ D if the patient survives it is best for the anaesthetist concerned to avoid being seen to check their progress on ITU or in rehabilitation
- ❑ E anaesthetists should inform their medical defence organisation following the unexpected death of any patient in their care

89 Management of continuous epidural analgesia in the hospital setting

- ❑ A epidurals can only be used for analgesia if the hospital has an acute pain service
- ❑ B there must be nurses with special training and skills in the supervision of epidural infusions available on the ward, on every shift, throughout the 24-h period
- ❑ C There must be 24-h availability of staff competent to recognise and manage the more serious complications of continuous epidural analgesia
- ❑ D aseptic technique for insertion of catheters should include use of a mask
- ❑ E the tubing between pump and catheter should have an injection port to facilitate top-ups

90 Intralipid in treatment of local-anaesthetic-induced cardiac arrest

- ❑ A is the first drug that should be given
- ❑ B the initial dose is 1.5 ml/kg of 20% intralipid
- ❑ C must be given into a central vein
- ❑ D is expensive
- ❑ E is contraindicated in people with anaphylaxis to soya bean

Practice Paper 2: The Clinical Vivas

Viva 1: The Clinical Viva takes place in the morning.

1. You are given a piece of clinical information and you have 10 min to study it.
2. You will spend 20 min with the first examiner, discussing the clinical care of the patient described and how you would anaesthetise for the case.
3. You will then spend 20 min with a second examiner discussing approximately three unrelated clinical scenarios.

Viva 2: The Clinical Science Viva takes place in the afternoon. Two examiners will question you for approximately 15 min each.

Approximately four topics are covered.

A good way to prepare for the viva is to work with a partner. For this reason we have separated the sample questions in this book from the model answers to allow you to work through the viva session before looking at the answers.

Viva 1

Clinical scenario
A previously fit and well 26-year-old primigravida at 32/40 weeks' gestation complains of increasingly painful paraesthesia of the thumb and index finger of her left hand.

Examination reveals pulse 100 beats/min, blood pressure 110/70 mmHg. There are first and second heart sounds plus a systolic murmur best heard in the aortic area. There is oedema of the legs bilaterally.

Laboratory investigations:
Hb 9.9 g/dl
WCC 11.9×10^9/l
Pts 156×10^9/l

Haemoglobin electrophoresis: HbA and HbS detected
Na 130 mmol/l
K 4.2 mmol/l
Urea 2.1 mmol/l
Albumin 29 g/l
ALP 356 IU/l (norm. 60–110 IU/l)
24-h urinary protein 150 mg
PT 12 s

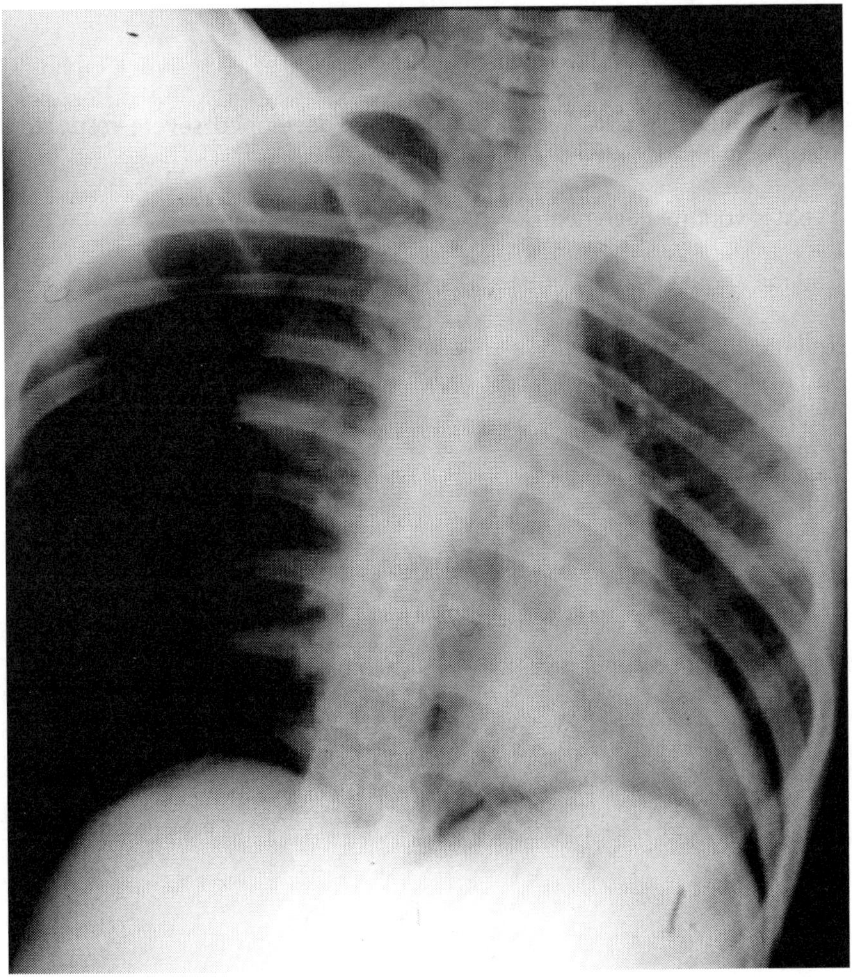

Fig. 4: Chest x-ray

Examiner 1
Summarise this case

What is carpal tunnel syndrome?

Comment on the physical findings and laboratory investigations

How would you anaesthetise this patient?

Examiner 2
What does this CXR show? (Fig. 4)

Shortly after this CXR was taken the lady developed severe respiratory distress, cyanosis and a barely palpable pulse

What is your management?

Tell me about eye blocks for cataract surgery

Tell me about the problems associated with acute 'ecstasy' intoxication

Viva 2

Examiner 1
Tell me about inotropes

Tell me about the problems of anaesthesia at high altitude

Examiner 2
Tell me about postoperative nausea and vomiting

Tell me about the predication of difficult intubation

Short Answer Question Paper 2 Answers

1 How would you preoperatively assess (40%), investigate (20%) and resuscitate (40%) a 6-week-old infant prior to repair of congenital hypertrophic pyloric stenosis?

Usually males, often low birth weight, presenting with projectile vomiting following feeds (though constantly hungry) at 2–6 weeks of age. Approximately 1 in 350 live births.

Assessment

A medical rather than a surgical emergency, effective preoperative rehydration and correction of acid–base abnormalities is the primary treatment goal and is the main factor contributing to the low operative mortality of 0.3% compared to 10% in the early 20th century.

- Hydration status.
  Vomiting produces dehydration and metabolic imbalance.
  Dehydration assessed clinically:
  (a) 5% loss, mild, dry mucous membranes
  (b) 10% loss, moderate, mottled cold peripheries, poor capillary refill, sunken fontanelle, oliguria and hypotension
  (c) 15% loss, severe, shocked and moribund.
- Metabolic imbalance.
  Loss of gastric hydrogen and chloride ions produces hypochloraemic alkalosis. Initially, the kidney conserves hydrogen ions in exchange for potassium but, with severe dehydration, sodium retention predominates in exchange for hydrogen, producing an acid urine. The end result is hypochloraemic, hypokalaemic metabolic alkalosis with compensatory hypoventilation.

Investigation

Blood tests reveal the metabolic abnormalities above, in addition there may be mild jaundice which is attributed to glucuronyl transferase deficiency, which develops as a consequence of starvation. An olive-sized mass may be felt to the right of the umbilicus and visible peristaltic waves may be seen in the upper abdomen after feeding.

The diagnosis is usually made clinically though ultrasound or endoscopy are sometimes used.

Treatment

- Preoperative resuscitation is essential. Surgery is not an emergency.
  (a) Nasogastric tube passed, aspirated frequently, nil by mouth instituted. Blood sugar should be monitored as hypoglycaemia may occur.
  (b) Intravenous fluid replacement. Saline (0.9%) with potassium supplements: initially 50ml/kg; 100 ml/kg or 150 ml/kg according to mild–severe dehydration and repeated according to response, electrolyte measurements and urine output.
  (c) Confirmation of resuscitation prior to surgery:
  Serum sodium > 135 mmol/l
  Serum chloride > 105 mmol/l
  Serum bicarbonate < 26 mmol/l
  Urine chloride > 20 mmol/l
  Urine output > 1ml/kg per hour.

Ref: Fell D and Chelliah S. Infantile pyloric stenosis. *Br J Anaesth CEPD Rev* 2001; **1**: 85–88.

2 What are the preconditions and exclusions for brain stem death testing? (50%) How would you perform brain stem death testing? (50%)

The preconditions for testing are:

- Apnoeic coma requiring ventilation
- Known cause of irreversible brain damage.

Patients must be excluded if:

- Hypothermic (core temperature <35°C)
- Central depressant or muscle relaxant drugs are present
- No severe acid–base abnormality or severe metabolic disease (eg profound hyponatraemia, uraemia hepatic encephalopathy)
- Uncontrolled endocrine disease (eg hypothyroidism or diabetes mellitus)
- Markedly elevated P_aCO_2
- Severe hypotension.

Brain stem function tests:

1. Pupillary reflexes – no direct or consensual reaction to light. Tests cranial nerve (CN) II and peripheral nervous system (PNS)

2. Corneal reflexes – no response to light touching cornea. Tests CN V and CN III
3. Oculocephalic reflexes remain in fixed position within orbit when ✗ head is rotated from side to side. Tests CN VIII
4. Caloric tests – after visualizing the tympanic membranes both sides, 30 ml ice cold water is injected into external auditory meatus. No nystagmus is seen if there is no brain stem function. Tests CN VIII
5. No response to painful stimulus applied to the face (usually pressure to the supra orbital fissure). Tests CN V and VII
6. Gag reflex absent during stimulation of oropharynx. Tests CN IX and X
7. Apnoea test – following ventilation with 100% O_2 patient is disconnected from ventilator (continuing passive insufflation of 6 l O_2/min). There is no respiratory effort during this time despite drive from a rising P_aCO_2. An ABG is taken to prove the P_aCO_2 is above 7.6 kPa. *(6.6)*

3 *A primigravid woman is found collapsed in the delivery suite following an epidural 'top-up' administered by the midwife 5 min before. List the likely causes (40%) and the initial management. (60%)*

Causes
- Aorto caval compression, impaired venous return causing low cardiac output.
- Intravascular administration of local anaesthetic, central nervous system toxicity causing convulsions followed by cardiovascular collapse.
- Subarachnoid administration of local anaesthetic causing total spinal.
- Other causes to which the temporal relationship to the 'top-up' was circumstantial (eg massive antepartum haemorrhage or amniotic fluid embolus).

Initial management
- Call for senior help: senior anaesthetist, obstetrician and midwife.
- Turn the patient onto the left lateral position or wedge to relieve any aorto caval compression.
- Assess the airway and breathing, control the airway if necessary by intubation and administer high-flow oxygen by face mask or IPPV.
- Assess the circulation, gain IV access with at least one 14-G cannula and monitor the ECG.
- Give IV fluids and vasopressors or inotropes to improve the circulation. If there is no cardiac output follow the advanced life support algorithms remembering that ventricular fibrillation following

intravenous bupivacaine is resistant to conventional therapy and may require bretylium.
- Send samples for cross match and send for emergency O-negative blood if uncontrolled haemorrhage is present.
- Frequently assess both the maternal and fetal response to therapy.
- Early discussion with the obstetrician of the mode of fetal delivery.
- After resuscitation take blood samples for toxicology including bupivicaine concentration in case of harm to the mother or baby.

4 A previously fit 30-year-old male sustains an isolated fracture of the femur during a motor cycle accident. Six hours after admission he becomes dyspnoeic. What are the likely causes and their initial management?

Possible causes
- Simple pneumothorax
- Tension pneumothorax
- Haemothorax
- Fat embolism
- Occult haemorrhage causing hypovolaemia.

Management
- Give supplemental oxygen while obtaining diagnostic CXR and arterial blood gas analysis, if the clinical situation allows.
- Assess the circulation and obtain IV access with large-bore cannula. Give fluid as appropriate. Clinically examine the patient for signs of a tension pneumothorax: markedly deviated trachea, hyper-resonant percussion note, absent breath sounds and cardiovascular compromise. If present this will require emergency decompression with a 14-G cannula in the second intercostal space, mid clavicular line even before a CXR is performed.
- Simple pneumothorax will require percutaneous thoracostomy tube while a tension pneumothorax will require a thoracostomy tube following emergency decompression.
- Haemothorax will require drainage via a thoracostomy tube, though this may cause worsened haemodynamic instability once the tamponading effect of the blood is removed. If there has been significant thoracic bleeding or a widened mediastinum on CXR cardiothoracic surgical input should be sought.
- Sources of occult haemorrhage, such as intra-abdominal, should be sought; these may require surgical intervention.

- Fat embolism syndrome will present with hypoxaemia and hypocarbia due to shunting of blood in the lungs which are obstructed by micro fat emboli.
- CXR may be normal, there may be a petechial rash over the trunk and conjunctivae; fat droplets may be found in sputum and urine.
- Management is aimed at improving oxygenation with supplemental oxygen or intermittent positive pressure ventilation (IPPV), and reducing on-going fat emboli. Early fixation of long bone fractures may reduce ongoing embolisation.

5 Describe your management of an adult patient brought into the accident and emergency department in status epilepticus.

Definition

A seizure or series of seizures lasting longer than 30 min without regaining consciousness. Mortality 2.5% and morbidity including focal neurological deficits, intellectual deterioration and chronic epilepsy make it a medical emergency.

Management comprises control of convulsion and investigation of aetiology.

Initial management

- Maintain airway, give high-flow oxygen via face mask, monitor vital signs – ECG, pulse oximetry and blood pressure.
- Gain IV access, give IV lorazepam 0.1 mg/kg (usually 4 mg dose).
- Obtain blood for analysis of blood count, electrolytes (including Ca), blood glucose, serum anticonvulsant levels and toxicology screen.
- Give phenytoin 15–18 mg/kg as slow IV infusion with close monitoring (may cause hypotension and dysrhythmias), and/or phenobarbitone.
- Give intravenous thiamine (250 mg) as Pabrinex if any suggestion of alcohol abuse or malnutrition.
- If seizures persist second-line therapy should take place on ICU as drugs used may cause hypoventilation, loss of airway reflexes and intubation may be required.
- Once intubated, sedation with propofol/opiate mixture without muscle paralysis so on-going seizures are visible.
- If on-going seizures third-line therapy of thiopentone infusion 3–5 mg/kg bolus followed by 1–3 mg/kg per hour with cardiorespiratory support.

- If continuing tonic–clonic convulsions compromise oxygenation neuromuscular paralysis may be considered with continuous EEG monitoring though EEG monitoring may not be available in all ITU situations.
- Investigation into aetiology: 25% of patients have idiopathic epilepsy; drug non-compliance causing status; 75% of patients have a brain lesion, metabolic derangement (commonly alcohol withdrawal), cerebrovascular lesion, drug intoxication (eg theophylline or tricyclics) or a space-occupying brain lesion.
- Differentiation will include both biochemical investigation and imaging via CT or MRI.

Ref: NICE-Protocol for status epilepticus 2003.

6 How may nutrition be provided for patients on the intensive care unit? (30%) What are the advantages and disadvantages of each? (70%)

There are two basic routes of providing nutrition for patients in the ICU: enteral feeding and parenteral feeding.

Enteral feeding

Provided via fine-bore nasogastric, naso-jejunal or enterostomy tube. Ideal feed is isosmolar delivered in a controlled manner to prevent gastric distension, usually over 18 h per day with a 6-h rest period.

Providing 1.5 g/kg per day protein and 32–40 kcal/kg per day as well as vitamins and minerals.

Advantages

Preferable, since cheap, physiological and protects gut from erosions via physical barrier and increasing splanchnic blood flow. Recent evidence suggests reduction in villous atrophy, incidence of nosocomial pneumonia and translocation of toxins across the gut wall.

Disadvantages

Requires an intact functioning gut (>25 cm of ileum needed). May be contraindicated with intra-abdominal pathologies (eg pancreatitis, post surgical bowel resection). Complications include: misplaced tube (there are now strict guidelines for testing the placement of nasogastric tubes using litmus paper prior to use), gastric distension and aspiration, diarrhoea, bacterial contamination of feed and variable absorption.

Parenteral feeding
Used in the absence of functioning gut. Provided as a hyperosmolar solution, administered into a central vein. Protein requirement assessed by monitoring daily urinary urea production, each gram of nitrogen is then matched by 100–125 kcal of energy.

Advantages
Variable absorption is not a problem. Can be used with a non-functioning gut.

Disadvantages
Complications are numerous, frequent and can be life threatening. Central venous cannulation has significant complications: sepsis of the line site and septicaemia occurs in up to 25% of patients. Metabolic derangements: hyperglycaemia, electrolyte imbalance (K, Mg, Ph), hyperlipoproteinaemia, hypercholesterolaemia, fatty infiltration of the liver are common.

7 **What are the indications for awake intubation in the adult? (30%) How may the airway be anaesthetised prior to intubation? (70%)**

Indications
- Anatomically deformed upper airway, especially if anaesthesia may lead to loss of that airway
- Inability to open mouth
- To avoid aspiration in patients with a full stomach
- Respiratory failure requiring ventilation, to avoid the cardio depressant effects of anaesthetic drugs.

Airway anaesthesia may be provided by several means
- Lignocaine nebuliser, 3 ml of 4% lignocaine over 10–20 min.
- Cocaine solution 4% (2.5 ml for 70 kg person) to the nasal mucosa. Superior laryngeal nerve block with a 23-G needle: 3 ml of 1% lignocaine is injected near the inferior border of the greater cornu of the hyoid bone bilaterally. Recurrent laryngeal nerve block by trans-tracheal injection of 3–5 ml of 1% lignocaine using a 23-G needle via the cricothyroid membrane. The oropharynx is anaesthetised either by sucking an amethocaine lozenge or by direct spray.
- Cocaine solution as before provides anaesthesia of the nasal mucosa. The fibre optic intubating scope is inserted and small amounts of 4% lignocaine are injected as it is advanced.

8 How may gas exchange and anaesthesia be maintained during rigid bronchoscopy? (70%) What problems are associated with each method? (30%)

Deep anaesthesia with spontaneous respiration

Classically children. Anaesthetic gases (usually oxygen, sevoflurane mixture) are delivered via the side arm of the ventilating bronchoscope. The vocal cords are sprayed with 2% lignocaine prior to passing the bronchoscope.

Problems

- Deep anaesthesia is required to tolerate instrumentation
- High resistance to breathing
- Both of the above may lead to hypercapnia and acidosis
- Anaesthesia will lighten when the eye piece is removed for biopsy/ retrieval of foreign bodies.

Paralysis and controlled ventilation

Methods of maintaining gas exchange during paralysis

- Apnoeic insufflation. Suitable for short procedures as P_aCO_2 rises 0.4 kPa/min. Intermittent ventilation to control the rise.
- Ventilating bronchoscope. Children especially may be hand ventilated using an Ayres T piece attached to the side arm of the bronchoscope. Changes in compliance or airway obstruction are detected easily but no ventilation when the eye piece is opened.
- Sanders injector. Injection of 4 Bar (400 kPa) oxygen via 16-G injection port.
  Obstruction to outflow will cause barotrauma; unsuitable for young children. Entrainment of variable amounts of air causing unknown F_iO_2.
- High-frequency positive pressure ventilation. Enables lower mean airway pressures with no air entrainment. High flow out of the bronchoscope risks debris being carried towards the operator.

Maintenance of anaesthesia in these cases tends to be via total intravenous anaesthesia (TIVA), commonly using a propofol/remifentanil mixture which provides good airway reflex suppression, rapid emergence and decreased pollution.

9 How would you diagnose, treat and investigate a suspected case of suxamethonium apnoea?

Prolonged paralysis may be caused by

- Reduced cholinesterase activity due to inherited atypical cholinesterase, reduced amount of cholinesterase (eg severe chronic liver disease or pregnancy) or inhibition of cholinesterase by drugs (eg ecothiopate).
- Excessive dosage; accumulation of suxamethonium and production of a dual block.

Management
- Maintenance of anaesthesia and oxygenation.
- Diagnosis of the nature of the block using neuromuscular blockade monitoring. With dual block there will be fade during the train of four and edrophonium will improve the fade whereas with prolonged depolarising blockade there is no fade (or more usually no response at all).
- Neostigmine has been used to reverse dual blockade.
- Spontaneous recovery, usually within 4 h, occurs with prolonged depolarising blockade, though there may be considerable variability in the duration of paralysis to as little as 30 min. This may be speeded by the administration of blood or plasma but spontaneous recovery is preferable.
- Following recovery, blood may be analysed for cholinesterase activity by the degree of enzyme inhibition by dibucaine or fluoride. (Normal dibucaine No 75–85, fluoride No 60.) Blood should be taken 24 h later for these tests.
- Atypical enzyme (0.03% population are homozygotes) dibucaine No 15-25 and fluoride No 20. Silent gene (0.001% of population are homozygotes). No plasma cholinesterase activity. Fluoride-resistant gene (0.0001% of population are homozygotes).
- Full explanation to the patient should be given with consideration of a 'Medi-Alert' bracelet and screening of other family members.

10 Write brief notes on the complications of blood transfusion.

May be classified into early or late, and immunological or other.

Early immunological
- Haemolytic immediate (ABO) incompatibility
    - IgM cold antibodies
    - In the awake patient, dyspnoea, chest pain and loin pain precede cardiovascular collapse
    - In the anaesthetised patient, hypotension, fever, and DIC occur

    - Reaction to leucocytes, platelets and plasma proteins causing fever and hypotension
- Graft versus host disease in immunocompromised patients

Early other
- Transfusion of infected blood: septicaemia from Gram-negative organisms (rare)
- Circulatory overload
- Air embolism, thrombophlebitis
- Metabolic: hyperkalaemia (rarely a problem) – potassium is taken up into cells as they rewarm; hypocalcaemia due to citrate toxicity only in massive transfusion; acid–base disturbance
- Coagulopathy: dilution of platelets and lack of factors.

Late immunological
- Rh incompatibility: IgG antibodies cause jaundice and haemolytic anaemia 7–8 days following transfusion
- May cause haemolytic disease of the newborn in rhesus-negative mothers

Later other
- Transmission of infection
    - Viral: hepatitis B or C, HIV, CMV
    - Bacterial: *Treponema, Brucella, Salmonella*
    - Parasites: malaria, *Toxoplasma*
    - Iron overload.

11 What are the options for postoperative analgesia following an open nephrectomy? (40%) State briefly the advantages and disadvantages of each. (60%)

Options broadly divided into systemic or regional.

Systemic
- Intermittent intramuscular opiate: technically easy, high safety profile, either on an as-needed (prn) basis or regular administration. Less safe if the patient is cold or peripherally shut down when variable absorption will occur. Involves difficulties with nursing delays, patient's reluctance to ask for analgesia, and peaks and troughs in plasma opiate concentrations with periods of inadequate pain control.
- Patient-controlled analgesia systems: involve use of high-tech pumps allowing the patient to control the amount of opiate required according to the level of pain. Patient must be able to understand and be physically able to operate the button. Side-effects of respiratory depression, nausea, vomiting and pruritis may be a problem.

- Systemic paracetamol may be used as an adjunct though non-steroidals are generally avoided acutely due to potential renal toxicity.

Regional

- Localised wound infiltration, variably effective and lasts a fixed period of time.
- Intercostal nerve blockade: usually performed at the time of surgery, during surgical exposure of the neurovascular bundle. Lasts a fixed period of time following surgery. A catheter may be left in situ for repeated boluses, however multiple blocks are necessary for full analgesia.
- Epidural analgesia: technically more difficult and invasive with complications (dural puncture, infection, hypotension) and requiring high level of monitoring to avoid potentially serious side-effects. Block may be ineffective or cause disturbing motor paralysis of the lower limbs.

12 What are the specific difficulties of anaesthetising an acromegalic patient for a transsphenoidal hypophysectomy?

Acromegalic patients pose a number of difficult problems:

- Tissue hypertrophy with an enlarged tongue and soft tissues will predispose to airway difficulties.
- Up to 50% of patients have obstructive sleep apnoea and may lose their airway on induction of anaesthesia.
- Co-existing disease is common: hypertension, left ventricular hypertrophy or failure and coronary artery disease occur frequently. Impaired glucose tolerance and diabetes mellitus occur in 25% of patients.
- Premedication. Continuation of regular medication, especially antihypertensives, may require insulin, avoid sedative medication if there is sleep apnoea, an anti-sialagogue may be helpful if a difficult intubation is anticipated.
- Intubation may require use of a fibre optic intubating scope. A flexometallic endotracheal tube is inserted to avoid kinking. May need a throat pack and preparation of the nasal mucosa using cocaine paste.
- Major haemorrhage may occur peri-operatively as the carotid artery traverses the carotid sinus near to the surgical field.
- Postoperative nursing on a high dependency unit with frequent neurological observations, close monitoring of blood glucose and

urine output. Diabetes insipidus is common and may require treatment with DDAVP.

Ref: *Current Anaesthesia & Critical Care* 1993; **4**: 8–12.

Multiple Choice Question Paper 2 Answers

1 Severinghaus electrode — Answers: D E

The in vitro carbon dioxide electrode (Severinghaus) is used to measure the tension of carbon dioxide in blood, P_aCO_2. The pH is what is actually measured; this is directly related to P_aCO_2 since:

$CO_2 + H_2O \leftrightarrow H_2CO_3 \leftrightarrow H^+ + HCO_3^-$.

CO_2 in the blood diffuses across a semi-permeable membrane. The above reaction then occurs at the pH-sensitive glass electrode, which is bathed in bicarbonate solution. The pH is measured, from which the P_aCO_2 is then calculated.

2 Monitoring of evoked potentials — Answers: A B C E

Evoked potentials are of very low amplitude (1–2 μV) and only emerge from the background EEG (amplitude 10–300 μV) after multiple summations. Auditory and visual evoked responses have been tried for depth of anaesthesia monitoring, and somatosensory potentials for the assessment of spinal cord function.

3 Helium — Answers: A B

Helium is stored as a gas at room temperature in brown cylinders at a pressure of 13.7 kPa (137 bar). It has a similar viscosity to oxygen, but is much less dense (density of oxygen is 1.3, helium 0.16). Its low density causes the voice changes seen when it is inhaled. Since density is an important determinant in turbulent flow, helium is useful in upper airway obstruction because of its low density, where flow is turbulent. It is, however, not of use in bronchospasm. Helium is non-flammable and does not support combustion.

4 Exponential process — Answers: B C E

The half-life is the time taken for the quantity of whatever is being measured to fall to half of its original value. The time constant is the time at which the process would have been complete had the initial rate of change been maintained. The time constant is longer than the half-life. After one time constant the original quantity has fallen to 37% of its original value and after three time constants 95% of the process is completed.

5 Microshock **Answers: A C**

Microshock is the term used to describe the delivery of very small currents (100–150 μA) directly to the myocardium, where they may cause ventricular fibrillation (VF). Microshock requires the presence of a faulty intracardiac catheter (eg CVP line) or pacemaker electrode touching the wall of the heart along which current can pass.

Saline-filled intracardiac catheters will conduct current, while 5% dextrose will reduce the hazard of microshock.

The severity of microshock is inversely related to current frequency so risk is greatest at low frequencies such as mains frequency and with direct current. Connecting intracardiac catheters to isolated (floating, non-earthed) power supplies reduces the risk of microshock.

Ref: Parbrook G D, Davis P D and Parbrook E O. *Basic physics and measurement in anaesthetics,* 3rd edn. London: Butterworth Heinemann, 1995, pp 213–215.

6 Mechanics **Answers: A B D**

Mass is fundamental, and so is scalar. Weight and acceleration are related to force, which, having a direction, is a vector. Kinetic energy = $\frac{1}{2}mv^2$ so doubling the velocity (v) increases the energy by a factor of 2^2 or 4.

7 Surgical lasers **Answers: A D E**

Different types of laser produce light at different wavelengths, and with different properties. Some can be used down fibreoptic cables, but not the CO_2 laser, which is readily absorbed by glass and water. Argon laser light passes easily through the eye, only being absorbed by haemoglobin in blood, making it ideally suited for ophthalmic surgery. Airway fires are a real risk, and reducing the combustibility of the gas mixture is one of a variety of sensible precautions.

8 Concerning the response of measurement systems **Answers: C E**

Drift is a variation in the reading which is not caused by a change in the measured quantity. Error which is dependent on whether the measured value is increasing or decreasing is termed hysteresis. Under damping results in oscillation and overestimation.

9 Concerning intra-arterial blood pressure measurement **Answers: A C E**

The important information is in the range 0–20 Hz (Hz is cycles per second). Cannulae are short and stiff to minimise damping.

10 In a positive (or upward or right) skewed distribution (such as might be found by asking a primary school class 'how many children live in your house?') **Answers: B D**

Most of the marks for this question rely on you knowing which way the skew goes. In the above example there will be a bunching of replies in the low numbers (one or two children in the house). The mode<median<mean. The mean is never the best descriptor of centrality in skewed data. A square transformation may normalise left-skewed data.

11 Carcinoid syndrome **Answers: B C D**

The carcinoid syndrome is due to the effects of serotonin (also known as 5HT), which is produced by a tumour, usually in the ileum. The syndrome only occurs in the presence of hepatic secondaries. It may lead to intermittent wheezing, diarrhoea and flushing as well as right-sided cardiac valvular lesions such as tricuspid stenosis. Medical treatment includes octreotide, ketanserin and cyproheptadine. Aprotinin (Trasylol®) may also be used, as it prevents the peripheral conversion of kallikrein to bradykinin, which some tumours secrete.

12 Nimodipine **Answers: A C D**

Nimodipine is a calcium channel blocker (less correctly called a calcium antagonist). Like all calcium channel blockers, nimodipine causes vascular smooth muscle relaxation, and therefore can cause hypotension due to a reduction of systemic vascular resistance. Nimodipine, however, acts preferentially on cerebral arteries and its use is confined to prevention of vascular spasm following subarachnoid haemorrhage. It is not a cerebral protector per se, however. It does not interact with aminophylline.

13 Constrictive pericarditis **Answers: A B E**

Constrictive pericarditis is characterised by a small heart on CXR, an elevated JVP, tachycardia, a low blood pressure and signs of right-sided heart failure. It may be due to tuberculosis, carcinoma, radiotherapy, rheumatoid arthritis or trauma. Usually there is an elevated JVP and ascites but no pulmonary oedema. There is pulsus paradoxus (an exaggerated fall in blood pressure on inspiration). The elevated JVP rises further on inspiration (Kussmaul's sign) and exhibits a rapid descent.

14 Aortic regurgitation **Answers: A B C D E**

The causes of aortic regurgitation are rheumatic fever, rheumatoid arthritis, bacterial endocarditis, hypertension, dissecting aortic aneurysm, syphilis, Marfan's syndrome, and the seronegative arthropathies including ankylosing spondylitis, Reiter's syndrome, psoriatic arthropathy and relapsing polychondritis.

15 Deep vein thrombosis **Answers: A B C D E**

DVT occurs commonly in the postoperative period. Pulmonary embolism, which may follow on from DVT, remains a common cause of postoperative death. The oral contraceptive pill increases the likelihood of developing a DVT. Pregnancy also increases the likelihood. Despite its name, the lupus anticoagulant is associated with an increased chance of developing a DVT. HbSC disease is particularly associated with DVT, especially during pregnancy. Polycythaemia and the other myeloproliferative disorders predispose to DVT.

16 Acromegaly **Answers: A B D E**

Acromegaly is due to hypersecretion of growth hormone from a pituitary tumour. Patients have coarse oily skin, prognathism, and a large tongue.

Arthralgia, glucose intolerance, hypertension and a thyroid goitre may occur. Hyperprolactinaemia may occur, leading to impotence, galactorrhoea, gynaecomastia and amenorrhoea in females. There may be hypercalcaemia and hyperphosphataemia with a tendency to form renal calculi. Progressive heart failure may be seen.

17 Diabetic autonomic neuropathy **Answers: A B C D E**

Diabetic patients are at increased risk of preoperative complications, mainly from autonomic nervous system (ANS) dysfunction. ANS dysfunction is associated with increased cardiovascular instability during anaesthesia. These patients generally fail to exhibit the usual pressor response to tracheal intubation and have a prolonged QT interval.

Profound hypotension, bradycardia and even asystole may occur during anaesthesia. Impotence, diarrhoea, incomplete bladder emptying and loss of sweat in the limbs are other manifestations of ANS dysfunction that may occur.

Ref: Raucoules-Aimé M and Grimaud D. Diabetes mellitus: implications for the anaesthesiologist. *Curr Opinion Anaesthesiol* 1996; **9**: 247–253.

18 Bleeding time **Answers: B C E**

The bleeding time is essentially a test of platelet and vascular function.

Vitamin K is required by the liver for the synthesis of clotting factors 2, 7, 9 and 10. A deficiency of this vitamin leads to a prolongation of both PT and APTT, but has no effect on the bleeding time. However, scurvy, due to deficiency of vitamin C, does prolong the bleeding time. This is because vitamin C is required for collagen synthesis. The defective collagen in the blood vessels in scurvy leads to a prolonged bleeding time. Haemophilia A and von Willebrand's disease are both inherited disorders affecting clotting factor 8. Factor 8 consists of several subunits.

In haemophilia A, factor 8c is deficient, leading to a prolongation of the APTT. In von Willebrand's disease, factor 8VWF is abnormal. Since this part of the factor 8 molecule is needed for platelet adhesion the bleeding time is also prolonged in addition to the APTT. In DIC there is consumption of clotting factors and platelets, leading to prolongation of PT, APTT and bleeding time.

19 Primary hyperparathyroidism **Answers: A B C E**

Primary hyperparathyroidism is most commonly caused by an adenoma of the parathyroid glands. It leads to demineralisation of bones with extra-osseous calcification, increased plasma and urinary calcium and renal calculi.

20 Papilloedema **Answers: A B C D**

Papilloedema is due to raised intracranial pressure. It is usually due to a space-occupying lesion such as a cerebral tumour or abscess. It can rarely be seen in cavernous sinus thrombosis, and with both occlusion of the central retinal artery and vein. It can be unilateral, as in the Foster Kennedy syndrome. There is optic atrophy in one eye, papilloedema in the other. It is caused by a tumour on the inferior surface of the contralateral frontal lobe. It can be seen with the hypercapnia of respiratory failure. However, in respiratory failure due to pulmonary oedema the P_aCO_2 is not usually elevated.

21 Blood cell antigen A **Answers: A C E**

The ABO blood groups are inherited in Mendelian fashion.

The ABO blood group system

Phenotype	Genotype	Antigens	Naturally occurring antibodies	Frequency (%)
O	OO	O	Anti-A, B	46
A	AA or AO	A	Anti-B	42
B	BB or BO	B	Anti-A	9
AB	AB	AB	None	3

O is universal donor

AB is universal recipient

The table shows the frequency of each blood type. The ABO blood group antigens are found on red cells, white cells and platelets and in the 80% of the population who possess secretor genes; they are also found in saliva, plasma, semen and sweat. Haemolytic disease of the newborn (HDN) is the result of damage to fetal cells by maternal IgG antibodies directed against fetal red cell antigens. Until recently HDN was almost always due to anti-D antibodies produced by a rhesus-negative mother who was carrying a fetus with rhesus-positive red cells. Since the introduction of prophylactic anti-D for rhesus-negative mothers the incidence of HDN has fallen dramatically and of the few cases that do occur most commonly it is due to anti-A produced by a mother of group O against the red cells of a group A fetus.

22 Obstructive lung disease **Answers: B C**

Obstructive lung disease (eg asthma) is characterised by a reduced FEV_1/FVC ratio and a reduced PEFR. Restrictive lung disease is characterised by a reduction in both FEV_1 and FRC resulting in a normal ratio. The TLCO (transfer factor), a measure of gas transfer, is made by assessing carbon monoxide uptake. Although a useful measure of lung function it is non-specific and can be reduced in many conditions including obstructive and restrictive problems.

23 Erythropoietin **Answers: A C**

Erythropoietin is made in the kidneys (85%) and the liver (15%). It promotes red cell production by the bone marrow. Production is stimulated by hypoxia or haemorrhage. Production is reduced in renal disease and accounts, in part, for the anaemia of chronic renal failure.

24 Rheumatoid arthritis **Answers: A C D E**

Rheumatoid arthritis is a systemic chronic inflammatory disease affecting up to 3% of women and 1% of men in the United Kingdom.

Although the brunt of the disease is borne by the joints, most of the organs are affected. In the cardiovascular system the pericardium, myocardium and endocardium may all be affected. There is often a normochromic normocytic anaemia. Renal failure may be due to analgesic nephropathy, amyloidosis or an autoimmune glomerulonephritis.

25 Phaeochromocytomata **Answers: A B C D**

Phaeochromocytomata are the tumour of 10s: 10% are bilateral, 10% are familial, 10% are malignant. The familial tumours may be associated with hyperparathyroidism, medullary thyroid cancer and pancreatic or pituitary tumours. They may secrete adrenaline, noradrenaline, dopamine, somatostatin and other neuropeptides. They may cause continuous or episodic hypertension, or hypotension. The adrenaline secretion causes hyperglycaemia.

26 Tidal volume increase **Answers: B E**

An increase in tidal volume is seen in renal failure and diabetic ketoacidosis. It is a physiological response to acidosis and is mediated by the peripheral chemoreceptors, located in the aortic and carotid bodies.

Ankylosing spondylitis is associated with a reduced tidal volume and a restrictive lung defect. In emphysema the respiratory rate may rise but the TV tends to stay the same or reduce. Cerebral haemorrhage usually causes respiratory depression.

27 Diabetic amyotrophy **Answers: B C**

Diabetic amyotrophy is a form of somatic neuropathy which causes wasting (usually of the quadriceps) and pain in the affected muscles. It is associated with an elevated CSF protein and responds to improved blood sugar control. Impotence and urinary retention in the diabetic may signify autonomic neuropathy.

28 Ruptured oesophagus **Answer: D**

The most likely diagnosis here is a ruptured oesophagus (Boerhaave's syndrome). This is usually caused by excessive vomiting. The patient complains of epigastric pain and there is surgical emphysema in the neck. Pulmonary infarction would produce chest pains and laboured breathing but no subcutaneous emphysema or epigastric guarding.

Similarly pneumothorax and ruptured trachea do not produce epigastric guarding. A ruptured diaphragm tends to produce shoulder tip pain as its innervation is from C3–C5.

29 Dystrophia myotonica **Answers: A C D E**

Inherited as an autosomal dominant gene, this condition, though rare, has implications for anaesthesia. The myotonia (delayed muscle relaxation following contraction) affects skeletal and smooth muscle. It may be precipitated by cold, shivering and suxamethonium and neostigmine.

Patients may have frontal balding with wasting of the sternocleidomastoid and temporalis. The disease is associated with low IQ, diabetes mellitus, gonadal atrophy, dysphagia, respiratory muscle failure and a cardiomyopathy. There is increased sensitivity to non-depolarising muscle relaxants and extreme sensitivity to opioids, barbiturates and volatile agents.

Ref: Russell S H and Hirsch N P. Anaesthesia and myotonia. *Br J Anaesth* 1994; **72**: 210–216.

30 Brown–Sequard syndrome **Answers: B C D E**

The Brown–Sequard syndrome is due to hemisection of the spinal cord.

There is ipsilateral spastic paralysis (upper motor neurone lesion) with contralateral analgesia and thermoanaesthesia due to destruction of the spinothalamic tract. Damage to the dorsal columns produces ipsilateral loss of vibration and joint position awareness and Rombergism (balance is worse when eyes are shut).

31 Blood gases in aspirin poisoning **Answers: A B C D**

The question is a little ambiguous!

In aspirin overdose there may be:
(a) respiratory alkalosis
(b) metabolic acidosis
(c) a mixed respiratory alkalosis and metabolic acidosis.

Salicylates, by stimulating the respiratory system directly, initially cause respiratory alkalosis. However, in overdosage they uncouple oxidative phosphorylation; consequent impairment of aerobic pathways superimposes a metabolic (lactic) acidosis on the respiratory alkalosis. Both respiratory alkalosis and metabolic acidosis result in low blood bicarbonate, but the pH may be high if respiratory alkalosis is predominant, normal if the two cancel each other out, or low if metabolic acidosis is predominant. It does not cause metabolic alkalosis, so the base excess would not reach +5.

Thus a pH of 6.9 is possible, but indicates a very severe overdose.

Equally a P_aCO_2 of 3.2 kPa would be possible, due to respiratory alkalosis. A P_aO_2 of 10 kPa is a normal figure for a healthy young adult breathing room air; there is no reason for the P_aO_2 to be deranged in salicylate poisoning (although during treatment fluid overload can occasionally cause pulmonary oedema).

32 Measurement of cardiac output by pulmonary artery catheter **Answers: B E**

There has been much controversy recently concerning the use of pulmonary artery (PA) catheters. A 1996 study in the *Journal of the American Medical Association* (*JAMA*) suggested that inserting a PA catheter led to an increased mortality in ITU patients and the authors asked the Food and

Drug Administration (FDA) to put a moratorium on the use of PA catheters, pending a prospective, double-blind, randomised study.

Ref: Soni N. Swan song for the Swan-Ganz catheter? *Br Med J* 1996; **313**: 763–764.

Ref: Connors A F Jr., Speroff T, Dawson N V, et al. The effectiveness of right heart catheterization in the initial care of critically ill patients. SUPPORT Investigators. *J Am Med Assoc* 1996; **276(11)**: 889–898.

Ref: Gattinoni L, Brazzi L, Pelosi P, et al., for The SvO2 Collaborative Group. A trial of goal-oriented hemodynamic therapy in critically ill patients. *N Engl J Med* 1995; **333(16)**: 1025–1031.

33 Treatments for poisoning — Answer: D

Oral methionine, or, more usually, intravenous *N*-acetylcysteine is used to treat paracetamol poisoning. Coma and respiratory failure are unusual in salicylate poisoning and assisted ventilation is thus rare. Dicobalt edetate is used as an antidote in cyanide poisoning.

Physostigmine may be used as a last resort in severe tricyclic overdose, where anti-arrhythmic agents have failed, but it may cause seizures, bradycardia and cardiac failure, and therefore is not generally recommended.

34 Prolonged intestinal obstruction — Answers: A B C D

Prolonged intestinal obstruction leads to dehydration and uraemia. The patient usually develops a metabolic acidosis and a compensatory respiratory alkalosis. The patient might well be hypoxic if only breathing room air, but there is no particular reason for hyperglycaemia.

35 Hypotension and elevated central venous pressure — Answers: A C D E

In haemorrhage the central venous pressure (CVP) is low, as is the blood pressure, since there is a reduced intravascular volume. In all the other situations listed in the question there is either pump failure (myocardial infarction, congestive cardiac failure), or obstruction to the pulmonary circulation (pulmonary embolism, tension pneumothorax). In these instances therefore the damming back of blood in the venous circulation leads to an elevated CVP, while there is hypotension due to the pump failure or the obstruction to blood flow.

36 Adult VF arrest — Answers: B D

For adult VF arrest, the first shock should be 360 J monophasic or 150–200 J biphasic. The first drug to be given is adrenaline in a dose of 1 mg intravenously.

Isoprenaline has no place in the management of VF arrest. It is used primarily in complete heart block while awaiting a transvenous pacing wire.

Intravenous bicarbonate is only considered after prolonged resuscitation, its use being guided by assessment of acid–base status. Bretylium tosylate at a dose of 5–10 mg/kg, although not a first-line drug, may be considered where the VF has improved refractory to DC shocks.

Ref: Resuscitation Council (UK) 2005

37 Acute spinal cord injury — Answers: B D

In acute spinal cord injury, suxamethonium is safe if given within 72 h of the injury. Steroids may be of some benefit in acute cord injury.

There is usually hypotension and bradycardia due to loss of the sympathetic innervation. Hypotension is undesirable as it reduces blood supply to an already compromised spinal cord.

38 Myxoedema coma — Answers: A C D E

Myxoedema coma is a medical emergency; mortality is about 50%. A patient with myxoedema coma looks hypothyroid, is hypothermic, hyporeflexic, bradycardic and comatose. Treatment should be in an intensive care unit and includes intravenous thyroxine (T_4) or triiodothyronine (T_3) as a bolus and then regularly for 2–3 days. If pituitary hypothyroidism is suspected then intravenous hydrocortisone is given to replace ACTH deficiency. Hypothermia is very common and requires active rewarming. Hypothermia can lead to pancreatitis, hypoglycaemia and ventricular fibrillation. Thyroxine (T_4) is given orally once the patient is stabilised. Either normal saline or dextrose can be given; the latter is used if there is hypoglycaemia.

39 Fat embolism — Answers: A B C D E

Fat embolism occurs with fracture or operation on a long bone. A triad of respiratory compromise, cerebral dysfunction and petechial haemorrhages may be seen. There may be a pyrexia and ARDS or DIC can supervene in severe cases. It is associated with a mortality of 10%–20%.

40 Convulsions **Answers: A C D**

There are many causes of convulsions that may affect the anaesthetist.

Among these are the metabolic causes such as hypoglycaemia, hypocalcaemia, hypomagnesaemia and hyponatraemia. Alcohol withdrawal, renal or hepatic disease and drug poisoning are all potential causes. Head injuries or intracranial pathology may be implicated.

Anaesthetic drugs (including ether, enflurane, ketamine and doxapram) may be the aetiology. Hypoxia is a potent trigger of convulsions.

41 Respiratory support **Answers: A B C D E**

A patient who is tired and sweating, with bounding peripheral pulses may well be in hypercarbic respiratory failure and require respiratory support. Use of the accessory muscles of respiration and a tracheal tug also suggest the patient is becoming exhausted and will require respiratory support.

42 Brain stem death **Answers: D E**

Before performing tests of brain stem function, two preconditions must be met:

1. The presence of apnoeic coma.
2. Irreversible brain damage of known aetiology.

Potentially reversible conditions that may mimic brain stem death (BSD) must be excluded, such as:

1. Alcohol, sedatives, muscle relaxants, poisons.
2. Hypothermia; the temperature must be > 35°C.
3. Acid–base disturbance.
4. Endocrine or metabolic disturbance; hypothyroidism or thyrotoxicosis, diabetic coma (either hypo- or hyper-glycaemia), hyponatraemia.

BSD is confirmed by the demonstration of the absence of brain stem reflexes. This must be performed by two doctors: one should be the patient's consultant. Both must be medically registered for >5 years; neither should be a member of the transplant team.

The tests are:

1. Fixed unresponsive pupils (pupil size is irrelevant).

2. Absent corneal reflexes.
3. Absent doll's eye movements (ie the eyes do not move relative to the orbit when the head is rotated side to side).
4. Absence of gag reflex.
5. Absence of vestibulo-ocular reflexes.
6. Absence of motor activity within the cranial nerve territory after painful stimuli to the head and peripherally. Limb movement may occur but is due to spinal reflexes and does not exclude the diagnosis of BSD.
7. Absence of spontaneous respiratory effort. During this test the P_aCO_2 must be >6.7 kPa (ie sufficient to stimulate breathing). Patients with chronic lung disease who rely on hypoxic drive should have a P_aO_2 of <6.7 kPa.

43 Causes of metabolic alkalosis **Answers: A B D E**

Metabolic alkalosis results from a loss of H^+ or K^+ or an ingestion of base. The causes therefore include vomiting, burns and poisoning. Cushing's syndrome leads to hypokalaemia. A gastrocolic fistula leads to loss of gastric acid, as does pyloric stenosis. Acetazolamide is a carbonic anhydrase inhibitor which may be used to treat metabolic alkalosis.

44 Disseminated intravascular coagulation (DIC) **Answers: A B C D**

DIC is a consumptive coagulopathy that may be triggered by many disorders. The result is consumption of platelets, fibrinogen and clotting factors with, paradoxically, widespread deposition of thrombus in the microvasculature of vital organs such as the kidney and brain. This thrombus activates thrombolysis and perpetuates the coagulopathy. The management, in essence, entails replacing what is missing, ie platelets, fibrinogen (cryoprecipitate) and clotting factors (FFP). Of relevance to the anaesthetist is the fact that it may occur in several obstetric situations including severe pre-eclampsia or eclampsia, amniotic fluid embolus and placental abruption. It may occur with haemolytic transfusion reactions, following prostatectomy and in any septic patient.

Ref: Baglin T. Fortnightly Review: Disseminated intravascular coagulation: diagnosis and treatment. *Br Med J* 1996; **312**: 683–687.

45 Acute liver failure — Answers: B C D E

Acute liver failure may be due to viral hepatitis (hepatitis A, B, C, CMV or EBV), alcohol, paracetamol or other toxins and, rarely (especially nowadays), halothane. The commonest cause in the UK is paracetamol overdose. Indicators of a poor prognosis include a prothrombin time $>3\times$ control, bilirubin > 300 µmol/l and a pH <7.3. The liver enzymes alanine and aspartate aminotransferase (ALT, AST) are characteristically elevated and are sensitive markers of hepatocellular damage.

46 Complications of tracheostomy — Answers: A C D E

The complications of tracheostomy may be early or late.

Early:
1. Bleeding
2. Pneumothorax
3. Cardiovascular collapse if hypoxia or respiratory acidosis is rapidly corrected
4. Surgical emphysema   Tracheal perf/Oesoph perf.

Late:
1. Infection
2. Tracheal stenosis
3. Erosion into cartilage, major vessel or oesophagus
4. Obstruction of tracheostomy tube

47 Left ventricular failure (LVF) — Answer: B D E

The pulmonary oedema of left ventricular failure (LVF) can often clinically resemble asthma. Both produce dyspnoea and wheeziness.

LVF is more likely to cause an elevated jugular venous pressure (JVP).

LVF is associated with pulsus alternans while asthma causes pulsus paradoxus. Both will cause hypoxia and resulting cyanosis. Both can cause wheeze on auscultation of the lung fields, but the wheeze is expiratory in asthma while there are classically fine, basal, inspiratory crepitations in LVF. While pulmonary oedema of LVF produces bilateral fluffy infiltration on the chest X-ray there are usually clear lung fields in the asthmatic's CXR.

48 Oxyhaemoglobin dissociation curve — Answers: A B

The oxyhaemoglobin dissociation curve position depends critically on the plasma concentration of 2,3-DPG. The P_{75} represents the oxygen partial pressure at which haemoglobin is 75% saturated with oxygen, ie venous blood. This is normally about 5.3 kPa (40 mmHg). The curve is shifted to the right (the Bohr effect) by decreased pH, raised temperature, raised levels of 2,3-DPG (as in chronic anaemia), altitude and hypoxia.

The curve shifts to the left in carbon monoxide poisoning, in the presence of HbF or other high-affinity haemoglobins. A rightward shift of the curve enables the tissues to extract oxygen from haemoglobin more easily.

49 Hypofibrinogenaemia — Answers: A C D E

In massive transfusion the level of platelets and clotting factors is reduced as stored blood contains no effective platelets and is deficient in clotting factors, including fibrinogen. A similar situation exists in disseminated intravascular coagulation (DIC) although the aetiology is entirely different. The oral contraceptive pill leads to an increase in fibrinogen, a hyper-coagulable state and an increased incidence of venous thromboembolism. Asparaginase, used in the treatment of childhood acute lymphoblastic leukaemia, causes hypofibrinogenaemia.

Prostate resection may lead to the release of procoagulant material into the circulation and a resulting consumptive coagulopathy.

50 Post abdominal surgery – complications — Answers: B C D

The patient is febrile, shocked (low BP and tachycardia) and has a low CVP. The likeliest explanation is that the patient is septic, which may be due to anastomotic breakdown, or pneumonia. Although tachycardia and hypo-tension are seen in myocardial infarction and cardiac tamponade the CVP is usually elevated. There is often a pyrexia associated with acute MI, but it usually peaks 3–4 days after the event.

51 Penicillins — Answer: B

The penicillins are bactericidal and act by interfering with bacterial cell wall synthesis. The most important side-effect of the penicillins is hyper-sensitivity, which causes rashes and, occasionally, anaphylaxis, which can be fatal. Ten per cent of patients who are allergic to penicillins will also be allergic to cephalosporins.

52 Chronic pancreatitis **Answers: A C**

Coeliac plexus block is the one most often used to treat the pain of chronic pancreatitis. It may also be used to treat the pain of pancreatic cancer. A stellate ganglion block is used to block the sympathetic innervation of the face and arm.

53 Soda lime **Answers: C D E**

Soda lime is used to absorb CO_2 in anaesthetic breathing systems. It contains approximately 90% calcium hydroxide. Sodium hydroxide (5%) and potassium hydroxide (1%) are present as catalysts for the reaction between soda lime and CO_2. An indicator dye is present to show when the soda lime is exhausted. In the most often used soda lime (Durasorb®) the dye is Clayton yellow, which turns from pink to yellow.

The reaction is:

$2NaOH + CO_2 \rightarrow Na_2CO_3 + H_2O$ and then:

$Na_2CO_3 + Ca(OH)_2 \rightarrow CaCO_3 + 2NaOH$

The reaction is exothermic and produces heat, sometimes up to 60°C.

One of the advantages of using low flow circle systems with soda lime is that the heat and water produced in the reaction help to warm and humidify the inspired gases. Soda lime is compatible with all the currently used volatile agents. Sevoflurane is degraded to Compound A in the presence of soda lime at elevated temperatures. While Compound A is nephrotoxic in rats there is no evidence of toxicity in humans. In the USA, however, sevoflurane is not licensed for use with soda lime at a fresh gas flow of less than 2 l/min. Carbon monoxide may be produced when certain volatile agents react with dried out soda lime. This may then lead to carboxyhaemoglobinaemia in patients.

54 Sevoflurane **Answers: All false**

Sevoflurane is a fluorinated ether and is structurally related to enflurane and isoflurane, but is not an isomer of isoflurane. It is isoflurane and enflurane that are structural isomers of each other. Desflurane, another recently introduced volatile agent, requires a heated vaporiser, as its boiling point is 22.8°C. While desflurane undergoes minimal metabolism (0.02%), sevoflurane undergoes about 5% metabolism. Sevoflurane is metabolised by the liver to produce inorganic fluoride ions. However, unlike enflurane, there is no evidence of renal toxicity from the fluoride ions produced by the metabolism of sevoflurane. Desflurane at >1 MAC produces a degree of sympathetic stimulation with tachycardia and hypertension. Desflurane has a MAC of between 6% and 9%, while the MAC of sevoflurane is about 2%.

55 Metabolic changes postoperatively **Answers: A B D E**

The metabolic and physiological changes that occur postoperatively are due in part to increased production of the stress hormones especially cortisol and the renin-angiotensin-aldosterone system. Cortisol antagonises the effects of insulin and causes hyperglycaemia. In addition it is catabolic and leads to protein breakdown and increased urinary nitrogen excretion. Both cortisol and aldosterone lead to retention of sodium coupled to increased urinary excretion of potassium. There is now much evidence to show that most patients experience quite profound sleep disturbances in the postoperative period.

56 Difficult intubation **Answers: A B C D**

There are many preoperative tests that are used to predict whether a patient is, or is not, likely to be difficult to intubate. Many of these tests yield a large number of false positives and, more worryingly, a significant number of false negatives too. Nevertheless a Mallampati grade 3 does suggest a difficult intubation, as does a reduced thyromental distance. While obesity is associated with difficult intubation, there is no such association with Parkinson's disease. The Wilson score is made up of five variables: weight, head and neck movement, the presence or otherwise of buck teeth, a receding mandible and mouth opening. Each variable is scored between 0 and 2 and a total score derived. A score of >2 suggests a difficult intubation.

57 Massive blood transfusion **Answers: A B D**

There are several definitions of massive blood transfusion including the replacement of the patient's total blood volume by stored homologous bank blood in <24 h. One of the greatest problems is the inevitable development of a coagulopathy, with thrombocytopenia and a prolonged international normalised ratio and activated partial thromboplastin time. This is readily corrected with FFP and platelets.

Cryoprecipitate may be necessary if the fibrinogen level is very low.

Disseminated intravascular coagulation (DIC) may occur in up to 30% of patients during a massive transfusion. Other problems with a massive transfusion include hypothermia, citrate toxicity, hypocalcaemia, hypokalaemia and a metabolic alkalosis. Pulmonary dysfunction may be caused by microaggregates in stored blood.

58 Acetylcholine — Answers: B D E

Acetylcholine is the neurotransmitter at all autonomic ganglia, postganglionic parasympathetic nerve fibres and the neuromuscular junction.

While noradrenaline is the neurotransmitter at most postganglionic sympathetic nerve fibres, the exception is the sweat glands. The adrenal medulla releases adrenaline and noradrenaline. The preganglionic innervation of the adrenal medulla is cholinergic.

59 Autonomic neuropathy — Answers: A C

Autonomic neuropathy is most commonly seen in diabetes mellitus, but can occur in AIDS, the Shy Drager syndrome (a variant of Parkinson's disease), and with bronchial carcinoma. The Valsalva manoeuvre is a standard test of the integrity of the autonomic nervous system (ANS). In ANS dysfunction there is no variation in heart rate during the test.

Normally there is a variation in heart rate with respiration; this is absent in ANS dysfunction. This can be demonstrated either on the ECG or by simple palpation of the peripheral pulse. Postural hypotension occurs in ANS dysfunction.

60 Antibiotic cover for patients with prosthetic heart valve — Answers: B C

The *British National Formulary* (*BNF*) contains guidelines for prophylaxis against endocarditis.

A patient with a prosthetic heart valve having dental work is considered a special risk and should receive IV amoxicillin 1 g and IV gentamicin 120 mg at induction; then oral amoxicillin 500 mg 6 h later. Patients who are penicillin allergic may have either vancomycin and gentamicin or teicoplanin and gentamicin or clindamycin alone.

61 Teratogens **Answers: A B E**

A teratogen is an agent that causes structural or functional abnormalities in the fetus, or in the child after birth. The most commonly recognised teratogens include thalidomide, the androgens, cytotoxics, lithium, retinoids and warfarin. Lithium can cause a hypotonic baby and in addition is associated with atrialisation of the tricuspid valve (Ebstein's anomaly). Warfarin should be avoided in the first trimester, when heparin should be used instead. Warfarin can be re-instituted from week 12.

Warfarin can cause fetal asplenia, rendering the neonate susceptible to infection with *Pneumococcus* and other organisms. It can also cause chondrodysplasia punctata. Carbamazepine may be associated with neural tube defects. None of the inhalational anaesthetic agents are teratogens. Although the tetracyclines can cause staining of the teeth in the developing fetus, they are not teratogens.

62 TUR syndrome **Answers: A B E**

The TUR syndrome may occur as a result of absorption of the irrigating fluid used. The volume absorbed is reduced if the height of the irrigating fluid is <60 cm and the duration of surgery <60 min. About 20 ml/h is normally absorbed. The fluid used is iso-osmotic 1.5% glycine solution.

As it is iso-osmotic its absorption does not cause haemolysis. Glycine is used as it has good optical properties without conducting electricity, thereby reducing the risk of burns. Glycine is an inhibitory neurotransmitter and thus its absorption causes CNS effects such as confusion, seizures, cerebral oedema and irritability. Absorption of large volumes of irrigating fluid into the vascular space leads to signs of pulmonary oedema and heart failure, often with hypotension and, paradoxically, bradycardia. Classically there is hyponatraemia due to dilution. The management involves giving oxygen, fluid restriction and possibly a diuretic. The serum sodium must be corrected slowly as too rapid correction may lead to central pontine myelinolysis, which has a very high mortality. Disseminated intravascular coagulation can occur as part of the TUR syndrome.

63 Ropivacaine **Answers: A B E**

Ropivacaine is an amide local anaesthetic agent. It is slightly less potent than bupivacaine, but has a similar duration of action. Its main advantages are that it has less central nervous and cardiovascular toxicity than bupivacaine and is more selective for sensory nerve fibres. Unlike bupivacaine, which is a racemic mixture, ropivacaine is a single enantiomer. Plasma protein binding of ropivacaine is slightly less than that of bupivacaine but the p*K*a is identical.

Ref: McClure J H. Ropivacaine. *Br J Anaesth* 1996; **76**: 300–307.

64 Recurrent laryngeal nerve **Answers: A B C**

The innervation of the larynx is derived from the superior and recurrent laryngeal branches of the vagus nerve.

The recurrent laryngeal nerve supplies:
(a) Sensory fibres to the larynx below the vocal cords
(b) Motor fibres to all the intrinsic muscles of the larynx, except cricothyroid

The superior laryngeal nerve supplies:
(a) Sensory fibres to the larynx above the vocal cords
(b) Motor fibres to cricothyroid

The recurrent laryngeal nerves are intimately related to the inferior thyroid arteries.

65 Lower oesophageal tone **Answers: A C**

Metoclopramide and cisapride are pro-kinetic drugs and promote gastric emptying. However metoclopramide is, in addition, an anti-emetic and increases lower oesophageal sphincter (LOS) tone. Atropine and morphine both reduce LOS tone. Domperidone is, like metoclopramide an antagonist at dopaminergic receptors. It also increases LOS tone.

66 Magnesium **Answers: A B C D E**

Magnesium has a number of properties that are relevant to anaesthesia.

It has effects at the neuromuscular junction, the CNS, the myocardium and peripheral vascular tree. It sits in the central core of the NMDA receptor. It is used as an anticonvulsant in eclampsia, as an antiarrhythmic and in the treatment of phaeochromocytoma. Hypomagnesaemia is seen in alcoholics, diabetic ketoacidosis and in patients taking digoxin or diuretics. It can cause tetany, seizures and prolongation of the QT interval leading to VT or torsades de pointes. Hypermagnesaemia is seen in Addison's disease, chronic renal failure and in patients on lithium therapy. Magnesium readily crosses the placenta and may lead to fetal hypotonia and respiratory depression.

Magnesium inhibits acetylcholine release from the neuromuscular junction and so potentiates the actions of the non-depolarising muscle relaxants.

67 Radial nerve palsy **Answers: A B D**

The radial nerve supplies triceps, brachioradialis and extensor carpi radialis longus. Hence damage to the nerve leads to paralysis of the extensor muscles of the forearm and hand, causing wrist drop. Pronation is a function of pronator teres, innervated by the median nerve. It is supination which is affected by radial nerve palsy. Because of nerve overlap there is usually only a small area of anaesthesia in a radial nerve palsy, confined to the base of the thumb. The thenar eminence is innervated by the median nerve.

68 Non-steroidal anti-inflammatory drugs (NSAIDs) **Answers: A B D E**

The NSAIDs act by inhibiting the enzyme cyclooxygenase, which is involved in prostaglandin synthesis. Prostaglandins sensitise peripheral nociceptors to the effects of substance P, histamine and serotonin. By blocking prostaglandin synthesis, the NSAIDs are analgesic. Prostaglandins are a group of compounds derived from arachidonic acid.

Arachidonic acid may be converted by the enzyme lipo-oxygenase to leukotrienes, most of which are bronchoconstrictors. Alternatively arachidonic acid may be converted by cyclooxygenase to cyclic endoperoxides and thence to either thromboxane (TXA_2) or prostacyclin (PGI_2). TXA_2 is produced by platelet cyclooxygenase and is a potent vasoconstrictor and platelet aggregator. PGI_2 is produced by vascular endothelium and is a vasodilator. In about 10% of asthmatics, especially those with atopic asthma, allergic rhinitis and nasal polyps, NSAIDs may precipitate bronchospasm. This may be due to the unopposed bronchoconstrictor action of the leukotrienes. NSAIDs may precipitate acute renal failure especially in elderly, dehydrated patients.

Prostaglandins are vasodilators at the renal afferent arteriole and thus NSAIDs may cause vasoconstriction, ischaemia and acute tubular necrosis. By blockade of TXA_2, NSAIDs inhibit platelet aggregation and may exacerbate surgical blood loss. In the gastric mucosa, prostaglandins have a cytoprotective effect and NSAIDs may cause gastric inhibition, peptic ulceration and even gastrointestinal haemorrhage or perforation. NSAIDs may be given with misoprostol, a synthetic prostaglandin, to prevent this side-effect.

69 Trigeminal neuralgia **Answers: B C D E**

Trigeminal neuralgia affects the 5th cranial nerve. It may be treated with carbamazepine, but may be intractable. It may, rarely, be a presenting feature in multiple sclerosis.

70 Etomidate **Answers: A B C D E**

Etomidate is a carboxylated imidazole. It is soluble, but stable, in water and therefore presented in 35% propylene glycol. It is eliminated by esterase hydrolysis in the liver and plasma. Etomidate depresses the synthesis of both cortisol and aldosterone by inhibition of the adrenal enzyme 11-beta hydroxylase. It has a low incidence of allergy and does not cause histamine release. It causes pain on injection, involuntary movements and there is a high incidence of postoperative nausea and vomiting. It is porphyrinogenic in animal models and is therefore probably best avoided in known porphyric patients.

71 Malignant hyperpyrexia **Answers: B C E**

Malignant hyperpyrexia is inherited as an autosomal dominant gene. The disease affects skeletal muscle and is characterised by episodes of muscle hypermetabolism. It may be precipitated by a number of anaesthetic drugs including, classically, halothane and suxamethonium, but not by nitrous oxide.

The local anaesthetic agents are all safe. Although previously thought to be associated with other muscle disorders such as Duchenne muscular dystrophy the only definite association is with central core disease. The disease is thought to be due to an abnormality of the ryanodine receptor which is the calcium channel in the sarcoplasmic reticulum of the muscle. Uncontrolled entry of calcium into the muscle leads to hyperpyrexia and muscle rigidity. The muscle damage that ensues leads to rhabdomyolysis, hyperkalaemia and acidosis. The only specific treatment is dantrolene. Diagnosis is by in vitro contracture tests on muscle using halothane and caffeine.

Ref: Halsall PJ and Hopkins PM. Malignant hyperthermia. *Br J Anaesth CEPD* 2003; **3**:5–9.

72 Air embolism **Answers: A B**

Air embolism may occur during posterior fossa surgery. It is detected by a sudden fall in end-tidal carbon dioxide on capnography. The treatment includes turning off the nitrous oxide and giving 100% oxygen. Nitrous oxide is much less soluble than nitrogen and will increase the size of an air embolism. Mannitol will help reduce cerebral oedema but is of no value in air embolism. Compression of the neck veins elevates the venous pressure and, together with flooding of the surgical site with saline, prevents further air entering the circulation. Lying the patient head down in the left lateral position keeps the air embolism away from the pulmonary artery and coronary ostium, by trapping it in the right ventricle.

73 Amniotic fluid embolism **Answers: A B C D E**

If amniotic fluid enters the circulation it produces sudden severe shock with respiratory distress and cyanosis. There is usually a raised CVP and widespread opacification of the lung fields. ARDS may develop. There is often a coagulopathy, usually DIC. The mortality rate is very high.

Treatment is supportive. A definitive diagnosis is usually made at post mortem, although fetal squames may be found in pulmonary artery blood if a pulmonary artery catheter is in place. There is some evidence that the more forceful uterine contractions are, as occurs with Syntocinon® infusion, the more likely amniotic fluid embolism is.

74 Cardioplegia **Answers: B C D E**

Cardioplegia is used for myocardial preservation while the aorta is cross clamped during cardiac surgery. Potassium is present in a concentration of 10–20 mmol/l. It causes depolarisation of the myocardial cells and arrest in diastole. Procaine is present as a membrane stabiliser, while magnesium reduces automatic rhythmogenicity.

75 Ankle block **Answers: B D E**

There are five nerves to be blocked in an ankle block: tibial, sural, saphenous, deep and superficial peroneal nerves. Apart from the saphenous nerve, which is a branch of the femoral, all the other nerves are derived from the sciatic. The tibial nerve lies behind the medial malleolus and deep to the posterior tibial artery. The sural nerve lies between the Achilles tendon and lateral malleolus. The saphenous nerve lies anterior to the medial malleolus. The superficial peroneal nerve lies above and medial to the lateral malleolus. The deep peroneal nerve lies between extensor hallucis longus and tibialis anterior and is lateral to the anterior tibial artery.

76 Neonatal airway — Answers: A C D E

The trachea is 4 cm long in the neonate; the narrowest part is the cricoid cartilage. The larynx is at C4 and reaches the adult position (opposite C5/6) at 4 years old. The epiglottis is U-shaped and the tracheal rings are not fully formed. The carina is at T2 (T4 in the adult).

77 Fallot's tetralogy — Answers: A B

Fallot's tetralogy accounts for 10% of all congenital heart disease and 50% of cyanotic congenital heart disease. It consists of a VSD, pulmonary stenosis, right ventricular hypertrophy and an overriding aorta. Clinical signs include clubbing and cyanosis and a murmur due to flow across the stenosed pulmonary valve. Syncope and squatting are often seen.

78 Morphine — Answers: A B D E

Morphine is an agonist at OP3 (mu), OP2 (kappa) and OP1 (delta) opioid receptors. These receptors have a number of sub-types. Stimulation of OP3 receptors leads to analgesia, euphoria, ventilatory depression and miosis (by stimulation of the Edinger–Westphal nucleus of the 3rd cranial nerve), bradycardia, inappropriate ADH release and reduced gastrointestinal motility.

Morphine can cause histamine release and nausea and vomiting (by stimulation of the chemoreceptor trigger zone). Morphine is metabolised in the liver to morphine 3-glucuronide (70%) and morphine 6-glucuronide (10%), itself a potent analgesic which is then renally excreted.

79 Retrobulbar block — Answers: All false

In a retrobulbar block, local anaesthetic is injected into the muscle cone thereby anaesthetising the ciliary nerves, ciliary ganglion, 3rd and 6th cranial nerves. A separate facial nerve block is required to paralyse the orbicularis oculi muscle. The lacrimal nerve, which controls lacrimation, sits outside the muscle cone and is not affected by a retrobulbar block. Enophthalmos and miosis are part of Horner's syndrome, due to loss of the cervical sympathetic supply to the eye. This is seen in a stellate ganglion block, not in retrobulbar anaesthesia. Although the intraocular pressure usually increases with a retrobulbar block, there is no rise in intracranial pressure and thus no papilloedema.

Ref: Berry C B and Murphy P M. Regional anaesthesia for cataract surgery. *Br J Hosp Med* 1993; **49**: 689–701.

Ref: Johnson R W. Anatomy for ophthalmic anaesthesia. *Br J Anaesth* 1995; **75**: 80–95.

80 Myasthenia gravis **Answers: B D**

Myasthenia is an autoimmune disease characterised by a high titre of antibodies directed against the post-synaptic acetylcholine receptor of the neuromuscular junction. It is often associated with a thymoma. Oat cell tumours are associated with the Eaton–Lambert syndrome.

Myasthenia may be treated by thymectomy, immunosuppression, plasmapheresis and anticholinesterases. There is increased sensitivity to non-depolarising muscle relaxants.

81 The following are standard induction doses for a 15-kg child **Answers: A B E**

Drug	Dose	×15 kg
Thiopentone	5 mg/kg	75 mg
Atracurium	0.5 mg/kg	7.5 mg
Suxamethonium	1–2 mg/kg	15–30 mg
Fentanyl	1 μg/kg	15 μg
Ketamine	2 mg/kg	30 mg

82 Foreign body inhalation **Answers: A B C D**

Foreign body inhalation is more common in children and objects preferentially go to the straighter and wider right main bronchus. It may present with obstruction of upper or lower airways, and is a differential diagnosis in chronic chest infections or cough. Chest X-ray may show collapse or, if the object is acting like a ball-valve, with over inflation. Removal is by rigid bronchoscopy.

83 Anaesthesia for patients who have transplanted hearts **Answers: A C D E**

Asepsis is vital in transplant patients as they are receiving immunosuppression; IV lines, ET tubes and laryngoscopes should all be sterile, and gowns and gloves worn. Denervated hearts do not respond to indirectly acting drugs such as atropine, and heart rate only responds slowly to circulating catecholamines. Myocardial ischaemia usually occurs without pain (angina) in denervated hearts.

84 Management of severe pre-eclampsia **Answers: B C D**

ACE inhibitors are contraindicated in pre-eclampsia. The platelet count is an accurate predictor of other abnormalities and if it is above 100×10^9/l there are rarely other coagulation problems. There are no large randomised controlled studies that show any benefit of colloid over crystalloid in pre-eclampsia (or in any situation).

85 Cricoid pressure **Answers: B C E**

The cricoid cartilage is at the level of C6. If there is active vomiting it should be released because of the risk of oesophageal rupture. Cricoid pressure often makes intubation more difficult, but it can sometimes aid in visualisation of the larynx.

86 Checklist for anaesthetic equipment **Answers: B D E**

The first thing to do is to make sure the anaesthetic machine is plugged in and turned on, followed by checking that the monitoring devices are on. Vaporisers only need checking at the start of a session or if they have been changed. Monitoring, breathing system and ancillary equipment (including tubes, scopes, suction) must be checked between each patient. The session check is recorded in the machine logbook. Checks of machine, breathing system and monitoring should be recorded on each patient's anaesthetic chart.

87 Platelet transfusion **Answers: A D**

Platelets are not indicated in stable patients, even ITU patients who are not bleeding or having invasive procedures, unless the count is $<10\times10^9$/l. They are not indicated to enable a neuraxial block if another technique is possible. Platelets are kept at 22°C in bags which are permeable to oxygen, factors which increase the risk of bacterial contamination and growth, particularly after 3 days storage (maximum storage is 5 days). A bag of platelets is either a pool of the buffy coat of 4 donors or from the apheresis of a single donor's blood.

Ref: *Blood transfusion and the anaesthetist.* Association of Anaesthetists, 2005.

88 Catastrophes in anaesthetic practice **Answers: C E**

Although unexpected deaths are rare most anaesthetists are likely to be involved with an anaesthetic catastrophe at some point in their careers, and even 'expected' deaths can be very traumatic. Bad news should not be broken over the telephone, but face to face with a consultant present. If the patient survives it is best for the anaesthetist concerned to be seen to take an ongoing interest by checking their progress on ITU or in rehabilitation. Failure to do so may paint a negative, uncaring, perception.

Ref: *Catastrophes in anaesthetic practice – dealing with the aftermath.* The Association of Anaesthetists, 2005.

89 Management of continuous epidural analgesia **Answers: B C D**

In the absence of an acute pain service a named consultant anaesthetist should be responsible for the supervision of acute pain management in the hospital. The epidural system between the pump and the patient must be considered as closed and should not be breached. The infusion systems must not include injection ports.

Ref: *Good practice in the management of continuous epidural analgesia in the hospital setting,* November 2004. Royal College of Anaesthetists.

90 Intralipid in treatment of cardiac arrest **Answers: B E**

Intralipid 20% is an emulsion of soya oil, glycerol and egg phospholipids, and is virtually identical to the solvent in propofol (although then at only 10%). It is used in the manufacture of TPN and costs <£20 for 500 ml. There are some animal experiments and case reports which suggest it may be useful in the treatment of local anaesthetic toxicity. The initial treatment of cardiac arrest is advanced life support as always, so oxygen and adrenaline are the first drugs used. It is isotonic, so can be given safely peripherally.

Ref: www.ucl.ac.uk/anaesthesia/meetings/Friday%20Morning.htm#

Practice Paper 2: Clinical Viva Answers

Viva 1

Examiner 1

Summarise this case
This is a previously fit woman in the third trimester of her first pregnancy who presents with carpal tunnel syndrome.

What is carpal tunnel syndrome?
Entrapment of the median nerve under the flexor retinaculum at the wrist. The median nerve subserves sensation to the thumb, index, middle fingers; motor to the muscles of the thenar eminence (except adductor pollicis) and the lateral two lumbricles.

Common causes include pregnancy, rheumatoid arthritis, hypothyroidism, acromegaly and amyloidosis.

Comment on the physical findings and laboratory investigations
Go through them systematically, explaining why they are normal in the pregnant state.

The murmur is most likely to be a benign flow murmur. Mild oedema is not pathological and that level of proteinuria is not indicative of pre-eclampsia.

How would you anaesthetise this patient?
A regional block is probably the technique of choice. The examiner will expect you to take him or her through exactly how you would perform, say, a brachial plexus block via the axillary route, including explanation and informed consent from the patient.

Further questions you should anticipate could include:
Comment on the electrophoretic findings
Would this influence your anaesthetic technique?
What local anaesthetic would you use?
What are the effects of a local anaesthetic on the fetus?
If the patient refused a regional block how would you manage this case?
What are the risks to both mother and fetus of general anaesthesia?

Examiner 2

What does this CXR show?
The CXR shows a large pneumothorax of the right lung. There is tracheal deviation and mediastinal shift to the left meaning the pneumothorax is under tension.

What is your management?
The clinical findings are those of a tension pneumothorax. This is a medical emergency and requires urgent decompression.
(1) Oxygen should be given immediately by face mask (as high F_iO_2 as possible).
(2) An intravenous cannula should be inserted into the right chest immediately.
(3) Once stabilised an intercostal drain should be inserted.

(This CXR shows the intercostal drain in situ with re-expansion of the lung.)

Ref. Harriss D R and Graham T R. Management of intercostal drains. *Br J Hosp Med* 1991; **45**: 383–386.

Tell me about eye blocks for cataract surgery
The two eye blocks commonly used for cataract surgery are:
(1) Peribulbar block: 2–5 ml of local anaesthetic is injected into the muscle cone just behind the globe using a sharp, short (25 mm) needle. The needle is introduced through the conjunctiva 2 mm away from the globe, midway between the lateral canthus and the lateral limbus. Akinesia is usually complete, but sometimes a further medial injection is necessary to complete the block by passing a 25-mm needle medial to the medial caruncle and advancing perpendicular to the face.
Any technique using a blindly placed sharp needle may result in serious complications threatening sight, including globe perforation.
(2) Sub-Tenon's block: 5 ml of local anaesthetic is introduced to the sub-Tenon's space through a small incision in the inferior nasal quadrant of the eye with a special curved and blunt-ended sub-Tenon's cannula. Posterior diffusion of the anaesthetic blocks sensation from the eye by direct action on the ciliary nerves as they pass through the sub-Tenon's space. Usually enough anaesthetic diffuses into the muscle cone to produce complete akinesia.

Ref: Carr C. Local anaesthesia for ocular surgery. *Anaesthesia and Intensive Care Medicine* 2004; **5 (9)**: 312–314.

Tell me about the problems associated with acute 'ecstasy' intoxication
Ecstasy is the street name for the drug 3,4-methlyenedioxymethamphetamine (MDMA). Taking the drug at 'raves' to facilitate prolonged and frenetic dancing may lead to dehydration and a syndrome similar to malignant hyperpyrexia with:

- hyperpyrexia
- muscle rigidity; trismus and bruxism
- rhabdomyolysis
- myoglobinuria and acute renal failure
- disseminated intravascular coagulation
- multiple organ failure
- obtunded level of consciousness
- seizures

The malignant hyperpyrexia treatment includes:

- rapid cooling measures
- IV dantrolene if temperature is greater than 40°C
- transfer to ITU
- control seizures
- support failing organ systems
- intubation and ventilation if necessary

Occasionally dancers have consumed vast amounts of water as prophylaxis against dehydration and have then died from water intoxication and the resultant cerebral oedema.

Ref: Hall A P. "Ecstasy" and the anaesthetist. *Br J Anaesth* 1997; **79**: 697–698.

Viva 2

Examiner 1

Tell me about inotropes
Inotropes are drugs which increase the force of contraction of cardiac muscle.

- Catecholamines increase cAMP and intracellular calcium. They may be endogenous or synthetic.
  Adrenaline – beta agonist, some alpha
  Noradrenaline – mainly alpha, some beta
  Isoprenaline – beta only
  Dopamine – alpha, beta and dopamine receptor agonist
  Dobutamine – selective beta 1 agonist

- Phosphodiesterase inhibitors
  Specific cardiac phosphodiesterase – enoximone
  Non-specific phosphodiesterase – aminophylline
  Both increase cAMP by preventing its degradation.
- Cardiac glycosides
  Digoxin alters the ATPase of the Na/K pump.
- Calcium
  Transient effect, increases cytosolic free Ca.
- Glucagon
  Unknown mode of action.

Tell me about the problems of anaesthesia at high altitude
There is low atmospheric pressure, although F_iO_2 is the same, the partial pressure is reduced. The need for greater F_iO_2 makes nitrous oxide a less potent anaesthetic.

Vaporisers
Saturated vapour pressure is unaffected, therefore the partial pressure of the volatile agent is the same. Because atmospheric pressure is reduced the delivered concentration is higher than that shown on the dial. Since anaesthetic action depends on partial pressure, not concentration, the same settings are used as at sea level.

Flowmeters
Since atmospheric pressure is reduced, a given amount of gas occupies a larger volume. Therefore a greater volume of gas is required to pass through the rotameter to maintain a given height. Therefore rotameters under-read. Since it is the number of molecules that is important, the rotameter is used as normal.

Examiner 2

Tell me about postoperative nausea and vomiting
Causes of postoperative nausea and vomiting (PONV) include
- Patient factors
  Females
  Young
  Anxiety
  Travel sickness
  Previous PONV
  Early mobilisation
  Eating and drinking

- Anaesthetic factors
  Gastrointestinal distension with gas, hypoxaemia, hypotension
  Drugs – opiates, etomidate, nitrous oxide
- Surgical factors
  Gynaecological surgery
  Ear and eye surgery
  Laparoscopic surgery especially around the stomach

Treatment of postoperative nausea and vomiting includes
- Systematic approach – drugs acting on the periphery (gastrointestinal tract), chemoreceptor trigger zone and the emetic centre
- Antidopaminergic, anticholinergic, antihistaminoid drugs
- The newer anti-5HT3 drugs
- Sympathomimetics

Tell me about the predication of difficult intubation
There are numerous tests but as the specificity of the tests is poor they will therefore detect many false positives.
- Mallampati test
  Grades 1–3
  Sensitivity 50%, specificity 96%
- Patil test
  Thyromental distance 7 cm
- Occipital–atlanto distance
  A reduction leads to inability to extend the neck at laryngoscopy
- Wilson's test
  Weight (>90 kg)
  Head movement
  Jaw protrusion
  Mandibular recession
  Buck teeth
  Score 0–2 for each. A score of >2 predicts 75% of difficult intubations.

Short Answer Question Paper 3

1. Describe your anaesthetic management of a 5-year-old who is bleeding following tonsillectomy 6 h previously.

2. How would you manage a severely head-injured patient during transfer to a neurological unit?

3. What is your choice of anaesthetic for a primagravid woman at 26/40 gestation requiring appendicectomy?

4. List the possible methods of measuring cardiac output. Describe one method used in intensive care.

5. What are the options for pain relief following a day-case circumcision of a 2-year-old?

6. What methods of monitoring are available to detect air embolism? Briefly state the problems associated with each method.

7. What are the advantages and disadvantages of the interscalene versus the axillary approaches to the brachial plexus block?

8. Write a letter to be carried by a patient who is thought to be susceptible to malignant hyperthermia.

9. Outline the specific complications related to laparoscopic surgery.

10. What are the causes of hypoxaemia in the first 24 h following surgery? (60%) How do you reduce its occurrence? (40%)

11. Outline the problems associated with anaesthetising a patient with sickle cell disease for an elective cholecystectomy.

12. How would you preoperatively assess a patient due for a left pneumonectomy for a bronchogenic carcinoma?

Multiple Choice Question Paper 3

1 A trial has shown that a new cardiac output monitoring device has reduced mortality in surgery for fractured neck of femur from 10% to 8%

- ❑ A the new device has reduced mortality by 20%
- ❑ B the trial is unlikely to have statistically significant results if there were 50 patients in each group
- ❑ C the trial is likely to have statistically significant results if there were 5000 patients in each group
- ❑ D the number needed to treat to avoid 1 death is 8
- ❑ E the number needed to treat to avoid 1 death is 100

2 Pulse oximeters

- ❑ A can cause burns to the skin under the probe
- ❑ B may be inaccurate in the presence of vasoconstriction
- ❑ C are inaccurate in the presence of pigmented skin
- ❑ D may be inaccurate in patients with tricuspid regurgitation
- ❑ E have a slower response time than transcutaneous oxygen electrodes

3 The measurement of oxygen in a mixture of gases may be made by

- ❑ A pulse oximetry
- ❑ B the Severinghaus electrode
- ❑ C a transcutaneous oxygen electrode
- ❑ D an infrared analyser
- ❑ E mass spectrometry

4 During magnetic resonance scanning

- ❑ A pacemakers are unlikely to malfunction
- ❑ B sudden asphyxia may result due to a quench
- ❑ C ferromagnetic objects may injure the patient
- ❑ D monitoring equipment may be affected by the magnet
- ❑ E ferromagnetic objects must be within the 50-G field

5 The gas laws

- ❑ A pressure × volume = constant
- ❑ B pressure × temperature = constant
- ❑ C the partial pressure exerted by a dissolved gas is proportional to the concentration of gas molecules in solution
- ❑ D Graham's law states that the rate of diffusion of gases is independent of their molecular size
- ❑ E the universal gas constant is represented by the letter n

6 Automated occlusive cuff blood pressure monitors

- ❑ A tend to under read at high blood pressures
- ❑ B tend to be inaccurate at very low blood pressures
- ❑ C calculate MAP as diastolic plus one-third of pulse pressure
- ❑ D do not require calibration
- ❑ E adult cuff width is 10 cm

7 Nitrous oxide can be measured by

- ❑ A infrared spectrophotometer
- ❑ B paramagnetism
- ❑ C quadrupole mass spectrometry
- ❑ D gas chromatography
- ❑ E Raman light scattering

8 The 'train of four' measurement of neuromuscular blockade

❑ A consists of four identical 0.2-ms stimuli delivered over 2 s
❑ B shows serial reduction in twitch height in the presence of depolarising muscle relaxants
❑ C when two twitches are detectable approximately 50% of the acetylcholine receptors are blocked
❑ D it is recommended that at least three twitches are detectable before attempting reversal of blockade
❑ E is painful for awake patients

9 Concerning temperature

❑ A the triple point of water is 0°C
❑ B at sea-level water boils at 373 on the Kelvin scale
❑ C rectal temperature is usually greater than core temperature due to bacterial fermentation
❑ D if atmospheric pressure is reduced to 50 kPa (0.5 bar) water boils at 80°C
❑ E the resistance of a thermistor decreases as the temperature increases

10 In transthoracic echocardiography

❑ A the normal range for left ventricular ejection fraction is 0.62–0.85
❑ B an aortic valve area of <2.0 cm2 = severe aortic stenosis
❑ C valve vegetations can only be visualised if they are larger than 2 mm
❑ D pericardial effusions are poorly visualised
❑ E pulmonary artery pressure can be estimated

11 Recognised complications of bronchial neoplasms include

❑ A hypercalcaemia
❑ B hyperkalaemia
❑ C inappropriate ADH secretion
❑ D Cushing's syndrome
❑ E hypothyroidism

12 A laboratory report reading as follows: serum sodium 127 mmol/l, serum potassium 6.0 mmol/l, serum chloride 85 mmol/l, serum bicarbonate 18 mmol/l, blood urea 18 mmol/l, fasting blood sugar 3 mmol/l is compatible with a diagnosis of

- ❑ A adrenocortical insufficiency
- ❑ B hepatic failure
- ❑ C renal failure
- ❑ D carcinoma of lung with inappropriate antidiuretic hormone secretion
- ❑ E high small bowel obstruction with vomiting

13 In a patient with head injury the following conditions necessitate surgery

- ❑ A persistent CSF rhinorrhoea
- ❑ B convulsions
- ❑ C depressed fracture of the skull
- ❑ D extradural haematoma
- ❑ E linear fracture of the skull

14 Serum creatine phosphokinase activity is characteristically elevated

- ❑ A 24 h after a myocardial infarction
- ❑ B in osteomalacia
- ❑ C in untreated thyrotoxicosis
- ❑ D in myasthenia gravis
- ❑ E in Duchenne muscular dystrophy

15 Carcinoma of the bronchus

- ❑ A may cause dementia
- ❑ B commonly results in a lymphocytic meningitis
- ❑ C may present with a peripheral neuropathy before the primary tumour is demonstrated
- ❑ D may cause cerebellar degeneration without metastasising to the posterior fossa
- ❑ E may cause superior vena caval obstruction

16 The ECG features of hyperkalaemia include

- ❑ A tall peaked T waves
- ❑ B delta waves
- ❑ C widened QRS complexes
- ❑ D U waves
- ❑ E shortened PR interval

17 Unconjugated bilirubin

- ❑ A is water soluble
- ❑ B does not cause kernicterus
- ❑ C is conjugated in the Kupffer cells of the liver
- ❑ D concentration in the blood in the neonate is influenced by the administration of phenobarbitone to the mother
- ❑ E is transported in the plasma bound to albumin

18 In Addison's disease

- ❑ A treatment should be with ACTH
- ❑ B the serum sodium is high
- ❑ C there is an inability to excrete a water load
- ❑ D there is hypertension
- ❑ E there is a metabolic alkalosis

19 Ritodrine

- ❑ A slows the heart rate
- ❑ B produces heart block
- ❑ C may cause pulmonary oedema
- ❑ D increases the force of uterine contractions
- ❑ E produces peripheral vasoconstriction

20 Ionised calcium

- ❑ A should be measured in a sodium heparin (blood gas) sample
- ❑ B may be measured in a 'clotted' (serum) sample
- ❑ C is affected by pH
- ❑ D falls during massive blood transfusion
- ❑ E is affected by changes in serum protein levels

21 Drug-induced hyperglycaemia may occur with

- ❑ A bendrofluazide
- ❑ B captopril
- ❑ C the oral contraceptive pill (OCP)
- ❑ D propranolol
- ❑ E prednisolone

22 In an infant suffering from persistent vomiting

- ❑ A bile in the vomit is compatible with duodenal atresia
- ❑ B the absence of bile in the vomit favours the diagnosis of pyloric stenosis
- ❑ C a plain X-ray of the abdomen is likely to provide diagnostic help
- ❑ D duodenal atresia is more likely if the child has Down's syndrome
- ❑ E rehydration and gastric aspiration should be undertaken before surgery

23 Transplantation of the ureter into the colon may result in

- ❑ A hypochloraemia
- ❑ B a reversible rise in the blood urea
- ❑ C hyperkalaemia
- ❑ D acidosis
- ❑ E hypoglycaemia

24 Dopamine

- ❑ A is a positive inotrope
- ❑ B can safely be given via a peripheral line
- ❑ C causes tachycardia
- ❑ D stimulates alpha and beta adrenergic receptors
- ❑ E crosses the blood–brain barrier

25 Clonidine

- ❑ A is an antisialogogue
- ❑ B may be administered epidurally
- ❑ C causes bradycardia
- ❑ D is an alpha-2 agonist
- ❑ E increases the minimum alveolar concentration of the volatile agents

26 Infantile pyloric stenosis is associated with

- ❑ A hypokalaemia
- ❑ B hyperchloraemia
- ❑ C metabolic acidosis
- ❑ D diarrhoea
- ❑ E polyuria

27 Causes of stridor in a child include

- ❑ A acute laryngotracheobronchitis
- ❑ B acute epiglottitis
- ❑ C inhaled foreign body
- ❑ D tonsillitis
- ❑ E bronchiolitis

28 Concerning neonatal physiology

- ❑ A the stroke volume is relatively fixed
- ❑ B low levels of vitamin-K-dependent clotting factors may cause haemorrhagic disease of the newborn
- ❑ C oxygen consumption is the same as in an adult
- ❑ D they are obligate nasal breathers
- ❑ E circulating blood volume is about 70 ml/kg

29 Regarding acute epiglottitis

- ❑ A the causative organism is usually viral
- ❑ B intravenous access should be secured before induction
- ❑ C extubation is usually possible in 48 h
- ❑ D it only occurs in children
- ❑ E antibiotics are of no benefit

30 Obstructive sleep apnoea

- ❑ A is caused by intermittent nocturnal lower airways obstruction
- ❑ B can be precipitated by alcohol
- ❑ C can progress to cor pulmonale
- ❑ D treatment may include uvulopharyngopalatoplasty
- ❑ E it is advised to premedicate with benzodiazepines preoperatively

31 In an unconscious patient the following clinical signs suggest a cervical cord injury

- ❑ A hypotension with bradycardia
- ❑ B diaphragmatic breathing
- ❑ C priapism
- ❑ D flaccid areflexia of the limbs
- ❑ E a fixed, dilated pupil

32 Intra-aortic balloon counter pulsation increases

- ❑ A left ventricular work
- ❑ B myocardial oxygen requirements
- ❑ C heart rate
- ❑ D aortic diastolic pressure
- ❑ E coronary artery filling

33 A patient with central dislocation of the hip following a motor car accident is noted to be shocked on admission, 1 h after the accident. The most likely cause is

- ❑ A ruptured bladder
- ❑ B blood loss
- ❑ C fat embolism
- ❑ D ruptured urethra
- ❑ E neurogenic shock

34 Signs of increasing intracranial pressure after head injury include

- ❑ A a decreasing Glasgow coma score
- ❑ B tachycardia
- ❑ C hypotension
- ❑ D small pupils
- ❑ E an increase in P_aCO_2

35 A patient brought into casualty is found to be gasping for breath and cyanosed. The trachea is deviated to the left and the right side of the chest is hyper-resonant to percussion. He immediately requires

- ❑ A a chest X-ray
- ❑ B an intravenous infusion
- ❑ C immediate needling of the right side of the chest
- ❑ D oxygen given by mask
- ❑ E determination of his acid–base state

36 In a patient suffering from chronic respiratory acidosis

- ❑ A there is increased renal excretion of bicarbonate ion
- ❑ B there is an increase in plasma bicarbonate ion concentration
- ❑ C the total buffering ability of the blood is not altered
- ❑ D there is a decrease in the renal excretion of hydrogen ions
- ❑ E there is an equal increase in the number of mmol/l of plasma bicarbonate and carbonic acid

37 Paracetamol poisoning

- ❑ A is associated with early metabolic acidosis
- ❑ B is associated with hyperventilation
- ❑ C regularly causes hypothermia
- ❑ D can be treated with N-acetylcysteine
- ❑ E has been successfully treated with methionine

38 Characteristic features of the oliguric stage of acute tubular necrosis include

- ❑ A the excretion of small amounts of highly concentrated urine
- ❑ B a progressive rise in central venous pressure
- ❑ C a high plasma urea with normal creatinine concentration
- ❑ D malignant hypertension
- ❑ E hyperkalaemia

39 After cardiac arrest

- ❑ A rapid defibrillation of ventricular fibrillation improves survival dramatically
- ❑ B calcium is indicated for asystole due to hypokalaemia
- ❑ C hyperglycaemia should be corrected with insulin
- ❑ D sodium bicarbonate administration may result in hyperosmolality
- ❑ E cooling may improve neurological outcome

40 Tetanus

- ❑ A may have an incubation period of over 20 days
- ❑ B may be prevented by the immediate administration of tetanus toxoid
- ❑ C may produce severe autonomic disturbances
- ❑ D should be treated with human antitetanus antitoxin
- ❑ E is more common with facial wounds than with wounds of the extremities

41 The meniscus level of a central venous manometer

- ❑ A is a guide to right ventricular preload
- ❑ B rises during the inspiratory phase of artificial ventilation
- ❑ C gives the most accurate readings when the catheter tip lies within the right atrium
- ❑ D should be measured against a previous base-line zero
- ❑ E will demonstrate a, c and v oscillations of the central venous pulse if the catheter tip lies within the axillary vein

42 In cardioversion for cardiac arrhythmias

- ❑ A the shock should be delivered on the upstroke of the T wave
- ❑ B general anaesthesia is not necessary if DC conversion with synchronisation is carried out
- ❑ C AC is safer than DC
- ❑ D no preoperative preparation is needed for elective cases
- ❑ E ventricular fibrillation may result

43 Ecstasy intoxication

❑ A leads to sympathetic overactivity
❑ B may be treated with dantrolene
❑ C is associated with renal failure
❑ D may produce Parkinsonism
❑ E may simulate eclampsia if it presents in pregnancy

44 The following may occur in hypothermia

❑ A a delta wave in the ECG
❑ B a metabolic acidosis
❑ C hypoglycaemia
❑ D a raised serum amylase
❑ E anaemia

45 In carbon monoxide poisoning

❑ A the pulse oximeter underestimates the oxygen saturation
❑ B the oxyhaemoglobin dissociation curve is shifted to the left
❑ C there is histotoxic hypoxia
❑ D the arterial oxygen tension is normal
❑ E the oxygen content of the blood is normal

46 An elderly man arrives in A&E. He is unrousable with a GCS of 6. Blood gases show pH 7.05, P_aO_2 8 kPa, P_aCO_2 3.2 kPa, bicarbonate 10 mmol/l, Na 135 mmol/l, K 4 mmol/l, urea 6, Cl 95 mmol/l and glucose 10 mmol/l

❑ A he may have taken an overdose of aspirin
❑ B he may have taken a methanol overdose
❑ C he requires intubation and artificial ventilation
❑ D this may be a case of diabetic ketoacidosis
❑ E the anion gap is increased

47 Overdose of cocaine

- ❑ A leads to excessive sympathetic discharge and increased sensitivity to catecholamines at peripheral receptors
- ❑ B the differential diagnosis includes thyrotoxicosis, phaeochromocytoma or ethanol withdrawal
- ❑ C the mainstay for therapy are sedation and cooling
- ❑ D phenothiazines may be used for sedation
- ❑ E ß adrenergic antagonists are used to treat cocaine-induced myocardial ischaemia

48 In acute pancreatitis

- ❑ A the majority of cases are necrotising which carries a worse prognosis
- ❑ B abdominal ultrasound is the radiological examination of choice to detect necrosis and peri-pancreatic fluid collections
- ❑ C high C reactive protein and LDH levels are found in necrotising pancreatitis
- ❑ D interstitial oedematous pancreatitis most commonly leads to multi organ dysfunction syndrome (MODS)
- ❑ E surgical resection of the pancreas is most often considered in necrotising pancreatitis

49 Concerning rhabdomyolysis

- ❑ A hypercalcaemia is commonly seen in early rhabdomyolysis
- ❑ B the absence of myoglobinaemia or myoglobinuria excludes the diagnosis
- ❑ C myoglobin causes direct renal vasoconstriction
- ❑ D alkalinisation of the urine causes reduced solubility of the Tamm Horsfall protein–myoglobin complex
- ❑ E the prognosis for myoglobin-induced renal failure is poor with less than 70% of survivors regaining intrinsic renal function at 3 months

50 Concerning electrocution

- ❑ A following high voltage AC shock asystole is the commonest initial arrhythmia
- ❑ B asystole may be primary following a DC shock or secondary to asphyxia following a respiratory arrest
- ❑ C creatine kinase levels are predictive of myocardial necrosis
- ❑ D following lightning strike extensive autonomic stimulation may occur
- ❑ E a vertical current pathway (hand to foot) is more likely to be fatal than a transthoracic one

51 A 12-year-old boy is to undergo elective surgery. His older brother died 2 years previously, following an anaesthetic. The parents were told that he died after developing a high fever. Preoperative investigations should include

- ❑ A a muscle biopsy
- ❑ B serum sodium
- ❑ C serum creatine phosphokinase
- ❑ D the fluoride number
- ❑ E plasma cholinesterase level

52 A patient develops oliguria after cholecystectomy. The blood urea was 10 mmol/l preoperatively, and is 33 mmol/l 2 days after surgery, with a urine osmolality of 300 mosmol/kg and urinary sodium concentration is 140 mmol/l. It is correct to state that

- ❑ A the preoperative blood urea of 10 mmol/l excludes pre-existing renal disease
- ❑ B the urinary sodium concentration would exclude renal disease
- ❑ C the urine osmolality of 300 mosmol/kg water suggests that dehydration and hypovolaemia are the cause of the oliguria
- ❑ D a normal response to stress is suggested by the urinary sodium concentration
- ❑ E the patient is dehydrated

53 The following features result from acute extracellular depletion of the body fluids

- ❑ A raised blood urea concentration
- ❑ B raised urine specific gravity
- ❑ C diminished skin elasticity
- ❑ D raised haematocrit
- ❑ E rise in urine osmolality

54 The use of large quantities of isotonic non-electrolyte solution for irrigation during prolonged transurethral resection of the prostate may result in

- ❑ A hyponatraemia
- ❑ B haemolysis
- ❑ C haemodilution
- ❑ D hyperkalaemia
- ❑ E hypercalcaemia

55 The right main bronchus

- ❑ A lies superior to the right pulmonary artery
- ❑ B is 5 cm long
- ❑ C gives off the upper lobe bronchus before passing posterior to the pulmonary artery
- ❑ D gives off the middle lobe bronchus which then divides into superior and inferior segmental bronchi
- ❑ E is a superior relation of the azygous vein

56 For the control of postoperative thyrotoxic crisis, the following are indicated at once

- ❑ A diazepam
- ❑ B digoxin
- ❑ C corticosteroids
- ❑ D propranolol
- ❑ E carbimazole

57 After partial gastrectomy the metabolic changes expected in the first 4 days include

- ❑ A hypoglycaemia
- ❑ B a reduction in the amount of sodium excreted in the urine
- ❑ C a decrease in the circulating free fatty acid concentration
- ❑ D an increased excretion of potassium in the urine
- ❑ E an increase in oxygen consumption

58 The following may relieve severe pain from osseous metastases of carcinoma of the prostate

- ❑ A orchidectomy
- ❑ B short wave diathermy
- ❑ C diethylstilbestrol
- ❑ D testosterone
- ❑ E radiotherapy

59 The carotid sheath contains the

- ❑ A common carotid artery
- ❑ B vagus nerve
- ❑ C internal jugular vein
- ❑ D sympathetic trunk
- ❑ E ansa hypoglossi nerve

60 During one-lung anaesthesia for a lung resection, the shunt equation predicts that the following may minimise the reduction in S_pO_2

- ❑ A hypoxic pulmonary vasoconstriction (HPV)
- ❑ B the application of PEEP to the dependent lung
- ❑ C clamping the dependent pulmonary artery
- ❑ D the application of CPAP to the collapsed lung
- ❑ E increasing the inspired oxygen concentration

61 Inhalation of 10% oxygen in nitrogen by a normal subject at sea level

- ❑ A if the minute ventilation is normal the P_AO_2 is about 6 kPa
- ❑ B if hyperventilation brings the P_ACO_2 to 1.5 kPa the P_AO_2 will be about 7.5 kPa
- ❑ C if hyperventilation brings the P_ACO_2 to 1.5 kPa the P_AO_2 will be about 5 kPa
- ❑ D there will be a fall in mixed venous oxygen concentration
- ❑ E if hypoventilation allows the P_ACO_2 to reach 6.5 kPa the P_AO_2 will be 1 kPa

62 With reference to colloids

- ❑ A 4.5% albumin solution has an oncotic pressure similar to blood
- ❑ B hetastarch can prolong the prothrombin time
- ❑ C polygeline can cause acute renal failure
- ❑ D dextran 70 alters red cell deformability
- ❑ E cryoprecipitate is rich in factor VIII

63 The following drugs may precipitate bronchospasm

- ❑ A aspirin
- ❑ B morphine
- ❑ C labetalol
- ❑ D ketamine
- ❑ E isoflurane

64 The signs of a porphyric crisis following anaesthesia are

- ❑ A weakness of the extremities
- ❑ B psychosis
- ❑ C respiratory insufficiency
- ❑ D renal colic
- ❑ E passing dark urine

65 Isoflurane vapour

- ❑ A concentration can be measured by using a refractometer
- ❑ B is less dense than nitrous oxide
- ❑ C will absorb ultraviolet radiation
- ❑ D can be measured by infra-red absorption
- ❑ E can be measured by the changes in the elasticity of silicone rubber

66 The following will raise the intraocular pressure in a normal eye

- ❑ A hypercarbia
- ❑ B acetazolamide
- ❑ C atropine
- ❑ D hypotension
- ❑ E respiratory obstruction

67 Perioperative hyperkalaemia can follow

- ❑ A intravenous suxamethonium
- ❑ B blood transfusion
- ❑ C intravenous calcium gluconate
- ❑ D intravenous sodium bicarbonate
- ❑ E major trauma

68 Nimodipine

- ❑ A is a calcium channel blocker
- ❑ B is cardioselective
- ❑ C is a hypotensive agent
- ❑ D is used for cerebral protection
- ❑ E interacts with aminophylline

69 Coeliac plexus block

- ❑ A may relieve pain in abdominal malignancy
- ❑ B may result in orthostatic hypotension
- ❑ C may cause impotence
- ❑ D may be used in the management of chronic pancreatitis
- ❑ E causes constriction of the sphincter of Oddi

70 Reactions to intravenous dextrans can be reduced by

- ❑ A slow infusion
- ❑ B giving simultaneous antihistamines
- ❑ C giving a test dose
- ❑ D using hapten dextran before infusion
- ❑ E giving it into a large central vein

71 The following drugs are absorbed transdermally

- ❑ A atropine
- ❑ B hyoscine
- ❑ C morphine
- ❑ D fentanyl
- ❑ E paracetamol

72 Propofol

- ❑ A is presented in 20% 'intralipid'
- ❑ B may cause green urine
- ❑ C has little effect on cardiovascular function
- ❑ D reduces ventilatory response to carbon dioxide
- ❑ E has no effect on intraocular pressure

73 Bupivacaine

- ❑ A is an amide
- ❑ B is highly protein bound
- ❑ C is contraindicated in malignant hyperpyrexia
- ❑ D may cause refractory arrhythmias
- ❑ E recommended maximum dose is 2mg/kg

74 Premature neonates

- ❑ A are prone to develop hypocalcaemia
- ❑ B are sensitive to non-depolarising relaxants
- ❑ C have reduced insensible water loss
- ❑ D have increased unconjugated bilirubin levels
- ❑ E are prone to develop hypoglycaemia

75 Ventricular ectopic beats occurring during anaesthesia may be treated with

- ❑ A lignocaine
- ❑ B verapamil
- ❑ C beta-adrenoceptor blocking agents
- ❑ D digoxin
- ❑ E carotid sinus pressure

76 Treatment options for pulmonary aspiration of liquid gastric contents of pH less than 2.5 include

- ❑ A bronchoscopy
- ❑ B bronchial lavage
- ❑ C diuretics
- ❑ D ventilatory support
- ❑ E broad-spectrum antibiotics

77 Synthetic oxytocin is preferred to ergometrine for intravenous bolus administration because it

- ❑ A causes less nausea and vomiting
- ❑ B is faster acting
- ❑ C is less likely to produce hypertension
- ❑ D causes less fluid retention
- ❑ E is longer acting

78 An obstetrician calls urgently for help because a previously undiagnosed twin has been trapped in the uterus following the injection of ergometrine. Under such circumstances the uterus can be relaxed with the aid of

- ❑ A thiopentone
- ❑ B suxamethonium
- ❑ C d-tubocurarine
- ❑ D halothane
- ❑ E salbutamol

79 Cardiovascular changes in pregnancy include

- ❑ A a fall in mean arterial blood pressure in mid-trimester
- ❑ B an increase in central venous pressure
- ❑ C an increase in heart rate
- ❑ D an increase in total red cell volume
- ❑ E no change in stroke volume

80 Concerning anaphylactic reactions

- ❑ A they are more common when drugs are given orally
- ❑ B serum mast cell tryptase is a sensitive diagnostic test
- ❑ C they are due to degranulation of neutrophils
- ❑ D isoflurane may relieve refractory bronchospasm
- ❑ E antihistamines may reduce the severity of a reaction if given before induction of anaesthesia

81 Cardiopulmonary bypass

- ❑ A venous drainage is under gravity via the left atrium
- ❑ B membrane oxygenators force tiny bubbles into the blood
- ❑ C defoaming is performed to remove traces of detergent
- ❑ D the arterial return is passed through 150- to 300-μm filters to remove debris
- ❑ E the pump prime volume is about 5 l

82 The maxillary nerve

- ❑ A the maxillary nerve is the second division of the trigeminal nerve
- ❑ B is a mixed motor and sensory nerve
- ❑ C enters the pterygopalatine fossa via the foramen ovale
- ❑ D the infraorbital branch supplies sensation to the upper molar teeth
- ❑ E may be blocked by an injection into the pterygopalatine fossa via an intra oral route

83 Anaesthetic management of a woman who is 8 weeks pregnant for open reduction and internal fixation of a forearm fracture

- ❑ A if general anaesthesia is planned a rapid sequence induction is always needed
- ❑ B nitrous oxide should be avoided
- ❑ C diazepam is a suitable premedicant
- ❑ D a regional technique is preferable
- ❑ E postoperative analgesia with paracetamol, diclofenac and PRN morphine is acceptable

84 Anaesthesia for repair of ruptured abdominal aortic aneurysm

- ❑ A a femoral arterial line is preferable to radial
- ❑ B as long as the cross-clamp goes on below the level of the renal arteries renal dysfunction is rare
- ❑ C overall mortality is around 20%
- ❑ D paraplegia is commonly caused by peri-operative CVA
- ❑ E epidural analgesia is vital for postoperative recovery

85 Anaesthetic management of post-tonsillectomy haemorrhage

- ❑ A if within 2 h of original surgery the patient can be considered as 'starved'
- ❑ B the blood loss can be estimated by weighing the swabs and bedding
- ❑ C agitated children should receive an inhalational induction before IV cannulae are inserted
- ❑ D delayed haemorrhage is usually due to infection
- ❑ E non-steroidal anti-inflammatory drugs should be avoided

86 Postoperative visual loss following non-ocular surgery

- ❑ A is usually attributable to prolonged pressure on the globe
- ❑ B occurs at a rate of 1 in 500 following spine operations in the prone position
- ❑ C blood loss is a risk factor
- ❑ D ischaemic optic neuropathy is the commonest diagnosis
- ❑ E visual function usually returns to normal over a few weeks

87 Electroconvulsive therapy

- ❑ A cannot be performed without the patient's consent
- ❑ B pre-treatment with an anti-cholinergic is advisable
- ❑ C the aim is to provoke clonic spasms lasting about 60 s
- ❑ D methohexitone is the most suitable induction agent
- ❑ E suxamethonium reduces the risk of long bone fractures

88 Transvenous temporary pacemakers for bradycardia

- ❑ A stimulate the myocardium of the left ventricle with a bipolar wire
- ❑ B the minimal stimulating current is determined with the pacing box in VVI
- ❑ C the minimal stimulating (threshold) current is usually about 1–2 mA
- ❑ D the pacing output should be set at 50% of the minimal stimulating current
- ❑ E when capture occurs the pacing box should be converted to V00

89 Desflurane as compared to isoflurane

- ❑ A causes more respiratory irritation
- ❑ B causes more respiratory depression
- ❑ C causes more cardiovascular depression
- ❑ D causes more coronary vasodilatation
- ❑ E causes more muscle relaxation

90 Increased levels of plasma unconjugated bilirubin occur in

- ❑ A haemolysis
- ❑ B Gilbert's disease
- ❑ C chronic liver disease
- ❑ D primary biliary cirrhosis
- ❑ E Dubin-Johnson syndrome

Practice Paper 3: The Clinical Vivas

Viva 1: The Clinical Viva takes place in the morning.

1. You are given a piece of clinical information and you have 10 min to study it.
2. You will spend 20 min with the first examiner, discussing the clinical care of the patient described and how you would anaesthetise for the case.
3. You will then spend 20 min with a second examiner discussing approximately three unrelated clinical scenarios.

Viva 2: The Clinical Science Viva takes place in the afternoon. Two examiners will question you for approximately 15 min each.

Approximately four topics are covered.

A good way to prepare for the viva is to work with a partner. For this reason we have separated the sample questions in this book from the model answers to allow you to work through the viva session before looking at the answers.

Viva 1

Clinical scenario

A 70-year-old lady presents for open reduction and internal fixation of a fractured tibia and fibula. She suffers with severe rheumatoid arthritis and in addition reflux oesophagitis. She wears a soft neck collar. She has had previous general anaesthetics uneventfully.

Her regular medications are methotrexate, diclofenac and omeprazole.

Clinical examination reveals severely rheumatoid hands but is otherwise unremarkable.

Investigations
Hb 8.9 g/dl
Na 140 mmol/l
MCV 69 fl
K 4.5 mmol/l
White count and platelets Normal
Urea 6.5
Creatinine 100
The ECG and chest X-ray are normal.

Paper 3 Clinical Sciences Viva Questions

1 Compare and contrast etomidate and ketamine?

In what situations would you use these drugs?

2 What is a laser?

What types of laser do you know and what are they used for?

What safety precautions are necessary?

3 Describe the anatomy of the lumbar plexus.

Describe how you would perform a lumbar plexus block.

4 Describe the effects mediated by the different types of adrenergic receptors. Give examples of drugs that act at these receptors.

The photograph is of lateral views of the cervical spine in flexion and extension.

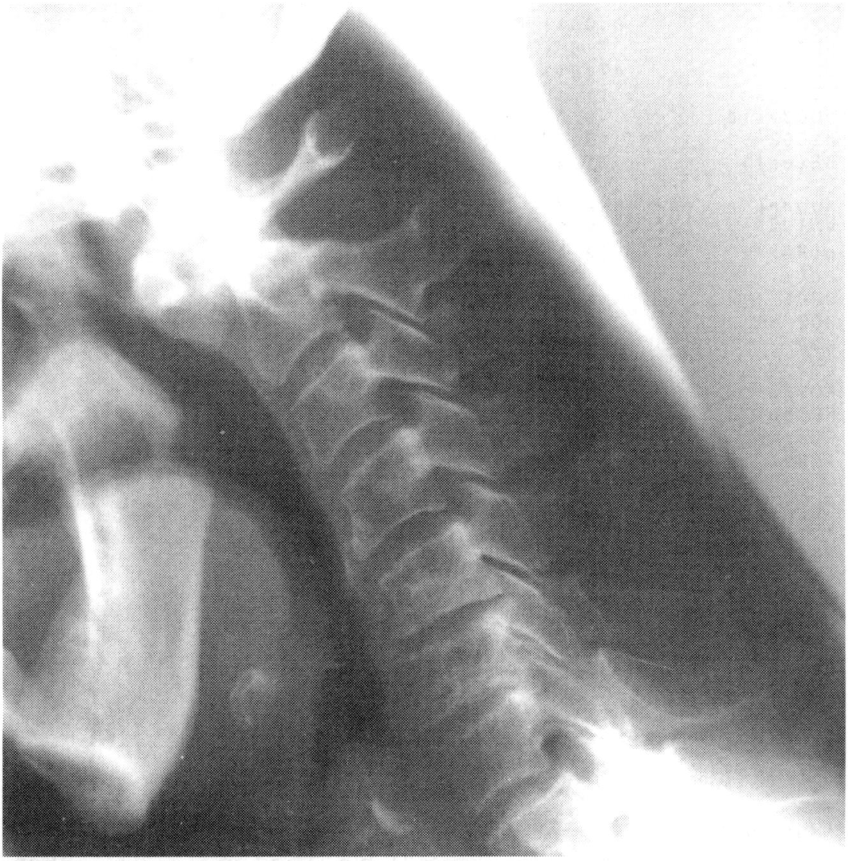

Fig. 5: Cervical spine X-ray

Examiner 1

Summarise the case and the possible anaesthetic implications

Describe the findings on the cervical spine X-ray. What is the significance?

How would you anaesthetise this lady?

SYRINGE SAMPLE

ACID/BASE 37°C

pH	6.904↓	
pCO2	7.86↑	kPa
pO2	47.84↑	kPa
HCO3-act	11.4	mmol/L
HCO3-std	9.0	mmol/L
ctCO2	13.2	mmol/L
BE(ecf)	-21.4	mmol/L

OXYGEN STATUS 37°C

ctHb	12.4	g/dL
Hct	36	%
O2CT	8.2	mmol/L
BO2	7.5	mmol/L
pO2	47.84↑	kPa
sO2	98.8↑	%
FO2Hb	96.1	%
FCOHb	1.8↑	%
FMetHb	0.9	%
FHHb	1.2	%

ELECTROLYTES

Na+	144.1	mmol/L
K+	3.29↓	mmol/L
Ca++	1.16	mmol/L
Ca++(7.4)	0.95	mmol/L
Cl-	101	mmol/L
AnGap	35.0	mmol/L

↑ or ↓ = exceeds reference range

Table 1: Arterial blood gases

Examiner 2

Here are a set of arterial blood gases (Table 1) and an ECG (Fig. 6) from a young girl of 16 brought into A&E by her parents having taken some tablets.

On arrival she is unconscious with widely dilated pupils. She is tachycardic and convulsing.

What do you think the diagnosis is?

What is your management?

The ECG (Fig. 6) was taken 30 min after her arrival in A&E.

What does it show?

What is your management?

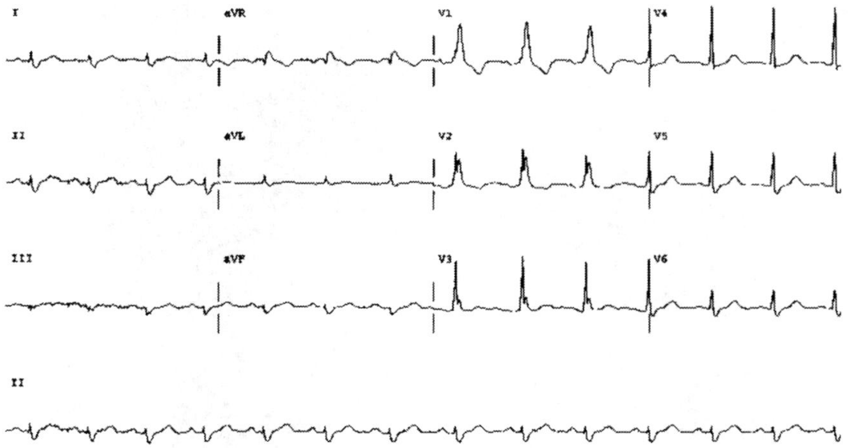

Fig. 6: Bifascicular block ecg

Viva 2

Examiner 1

Here is a PA and lateral chest X-ray (Figs. 7 and 8) of a woman in her 60s presenting for routine orthopaedic surgery. She has never had a previous anaesthetic but takes tablets for weakness.

What does the chest X-ray show?

What is the likely underlying diagnosis?

What is myasthenia gravis?

What medications and other treatments are there for this condition?

What are the anaesthetic implications of myasthenia gravis?

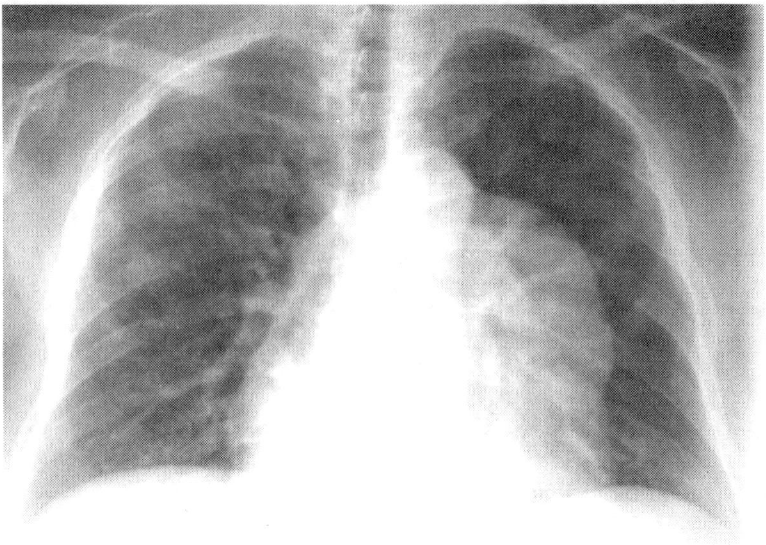

Fig. 7: PA X-ray

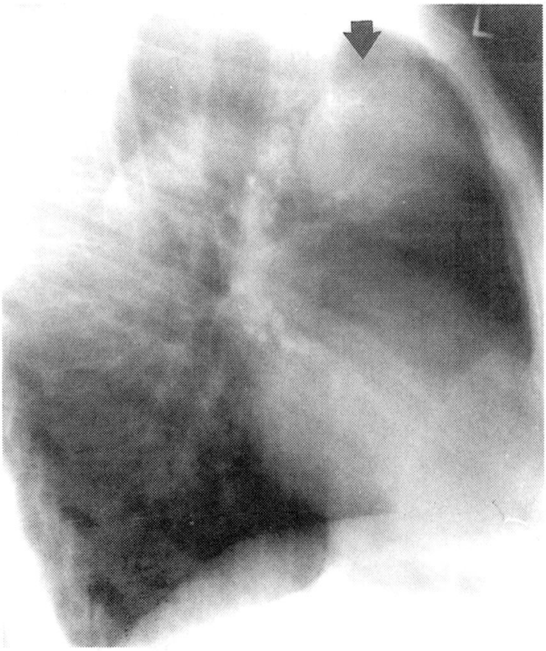

Fig. 8: Lateral X-ray

Examiner 2

Here is a CT scan (Fig. 9) of the brain of a young man who presented to A&E having been knocked unconscious playing rugby. He was initially lucid after regaining consciousness but then lapsed into coma.

What does the scan show?

Describe your initial management of this man in A&E.

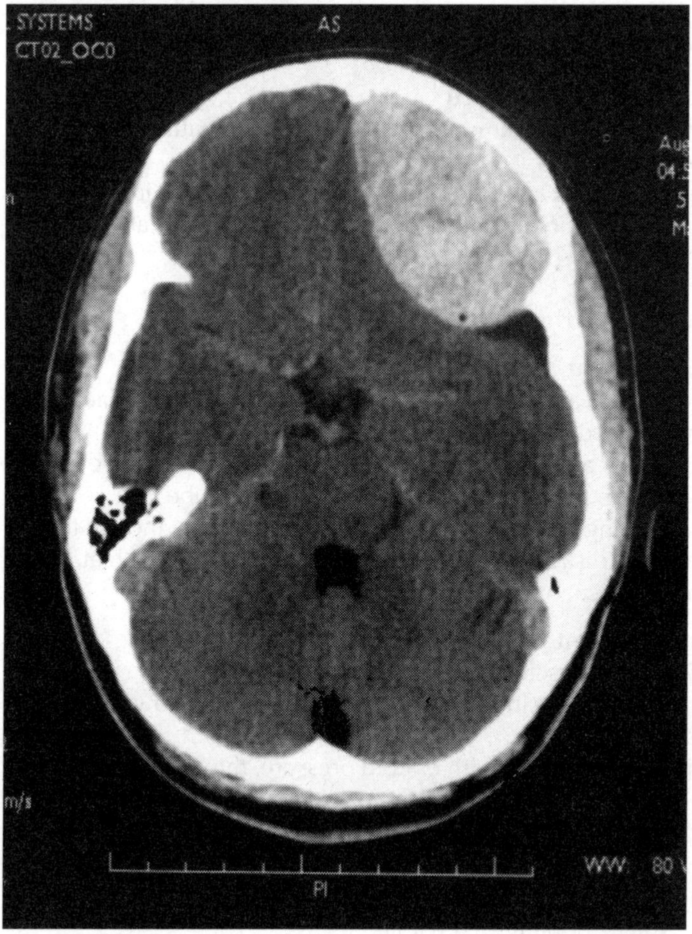

Fig. 9: CT scan

Describe your anaesthetic management of a five-year-old who is bleeding following tonsillectomy 6 h previously.

Short Answer Question Paper 3 Answers

1. **Describe your anaesthetic management of a 5-year-old who is bleeding following tonsillectomy 6 h previously.**

Problems which must be addressed

- Haemorrhage – often the amount is underestimated with possible hypovolaemia
- Swallowed blood and a full stomach predispose to aspiration
- Potentially difficult airway with blood obscuring the view at laryngoscopy
- Residual anaesthetic
- Frightened child and anxious parents.

Preoperative assessment

- Intravenous access and fluid replacement to ensure normovolaemia with cross-matched blood available
- Establish whether any anaesthetic difficulties were encountered at the original operation, noting particularly endotracheal tube size
- Consider emptying the stomach with a nasogastric tube, though this may cause more distress and bleeding; or premedication with atropine and an anti-emetic.

Anaesthetic management

- Ensure adequate resuscitation prior to induction
- Full monitoring prior to induction on tilting table head down, with effective suction
- Rapid sequence induction with cricoid pressure, thiopentone and suxamethonium
- Endotracheal intubation which may require a smaller sized tube than before
- Maintenance with air, oxygen and isoflurane, spontaneously breathing through a T-piece or paralysed with IPPV
- Prior to extubation wash the stomach out via a nasogastric tube inserted under direct vision by the surgeon to reduce possibility of causing further haemorrhage
- Extubate head down on side, fully awake.

Postoperatively
- Check Hb
- Beware of airway obstruction if the throat has been packed or if pre-existing sleep apnoea
- Consider high dependency unit for close monitoring.

2. How would you manage a severely head-injured patient during transfer to a neurological unit?

Problems to be addressed
- Potentially unstable patient, transferred in isolated environment with limited equipment and personnel
- Continuation of therapy to avoid secondary brain injury
- Prior to transfer it may be indicated to intubate patient (if not already intubated) especially if a fluctuating level of consciousness, swelling or bleeding from face injuries may make intubation more difficult, or seizures (remember cervical spine control during intubation)
- Associated injuries (present in 30%) sought and managed prior to transfer
- Adequate resuscitation of any associated injuries
- Appropriate personnel – at least one trained assistant
- Equipment appropriate to patient – including ventilator, oxygen and reserve drugs, fluids and blood, as well as alternative method of ventilation (Ambu-bag) should ventilator oxygen fail
- Appropriate mobile monitoring available including ECG, invasive pressure and pulse oximetry.

Continuation of therapy to avoid secondary brain injury
- Ensure adequate flux of oxygen to brain tissue with impaired autoregulation
- High inspired oxygen
- Ensure mean arterial pressure adequate to perfuse brain despite rising intracranial pressure – by use of fluids and/or inotropes
- Aim to limit rising intracranial pressure (this may only be possible by definitive neurosurgical intervention)
- Moderate hyperventilation to P_aCO_2 4–4.5 kPa
- Avoid straining, coughing
- Avoid tight endotracheal ties, venous congestion
- Ensure adequate sedation prior to movement or intervention (eg suctioning), consider mannitol if acute deterioration (unilateral increase in pupil size)

- Careful continued monitoring including invasive blood pressure, ECG, P_aO_2 and ET CO_2 together with frequent clinical evaluation – pupil size in paralysed, ventilated patient
- Glasgow coma scale in un-intubated patient.

Ref: Association of Anaesthetists of Great Britain and Ireland. *Recommendations for the safe transfer of patients with a head injury*. 2006. Available online at http://www.aagbi.org/publications/guidelines/docs/brain_injury.pdf

3. What is your choice of anaesthetic for a primagravid woman at 26/40 gestation requiring appendicectomy?

General considerations

- Safe anaesthesia for the woman, remembering increased blood volume and cardiac output. Increased oxygen consumption together with reduced functional residual capacity and pulmonary compliance lead to early desaturation.
- Fetal considerations: maintaining placental blood flow and avoidance of teratogens.

Preoperative management

- Thorough assessment, particularly airway; may need rehydration with intravenous fluids
- Acid aspiration prophylaxis, ranitidine and sodium citrate
- Liaise with obstetric staff for fetal monitoring pre- and postoperative
- Avoid aortocaval compression, transportation in left lateral position
- Graduated compression stockings advisable as hypercoagulability and venous stasis predispose to thromboembolism
- Rapid sequence induction and intubation with pre-oxygenation, 15° lateral tilt and cricoid pressure using thiopentone and suxamethonium (no anaesthetic drugs have been conclusively proven to be safe or teratogenic)
- Maintenance using IPPV, relaxant, oxygen and volatile agent with supplemental opioid
- Extubation in left lateral position, fully awake, ensure good oxygenation and continue fetal monitoring
- Analgesia provided by opioids often using patient-controlled analgesia system
- Avoidance of non-steroidal anti-inflammatory drugs due to the theoretical risk of premature ductus closure in utero.

4. List the possible methods of measuring cardiac output. Describe one method used in intensive care.

Cardiac output: the volume of blood pumped by the heart per minute.

- Fick principle: usually oxygen consumption is measured. Requires samples of arterial and mixed venous blood to calculate their oxygen content.
  O_2 consumption = (arterial – mixed venous O_2 concentration) × cardiac output
- Dilutional techniques: either dye or cold saline is used as the indicator.
- Transoesophageal echocardiography using the Doppler effect: the velocity of blood in the descending aorta is measured, which, when multiplied by the aortic cross-sectional area, gives the stroke volume.
- Cardiac catheterisation: highly invasive, giving an estimate of stroke volume.
- Radioisotope scanning: gives an average stroke volume over a long time period. Unsuitable for rapid variations.
- Echocardiography: two-dimensional view gives an estimate of stroke volume. Large inter-operator variability.
- Impedance plethysmography: a research tool.

Dilutional techniques

- Most commonly used in intensive care. Requires pulmonary artery catheterisation.
- Cold saline is used as the indicator for repeated measurements. A thermistor situated at the catheter tip measures the change in temperature.
- 5–10 ml of saline is injected at end expiration into the proximal port (RA) of the pulmonary artery catheter.
- The change in temperature of blood passing through the pulmonary artery is detected against time. A semi-logarithmic plot is made: temperature change against time. The area under the curve gives the cardiac output.
- The average of three measurements is taken.
- Cold water indicator avoids the second peak of dye recirculation and allows repeated measurements in critically ill patients.

5. What are the options for pain relief following day-case circumcision in a 2-year-old?

- Requirement for adequate analgesia with low incidence of side-effects.

- The variable response of children to opiate analgesics with potential for serious side-effects of sedation and respiratory depression makes them less useful in day-case settings.
- Non-steroidal drugs are a useful adjunct though insufficient alone. Unsuitable for children with asthma as they may precipitate bronchospasm.
- Regional techniques are popular, providing local analgesia with minimal side-effects.
  (a) Penile block. Dorsal nerves of the penis derive from the pudendal nerve. May be blocked by injection of 2–5 ml of 0.25% plain bupivacaine inferior to the symphysis pubis in the mid line below Buck's fascia. Genital branch of the genitofemoral nerve blocked separately by subcutaneous infiltration on the ventral surface of the penis. Good quality analgesia, few side-effects: haematoma, misplacement of solution, urinary retention unlikely.
  (b) Caudal analgesia. Bupivacaine (0.5 ml/kg of 0.25%) injected through sacrococcygeal membrane. Provides good quality analgesia but frequent side-effects: urinary retention and weakness of lower limbs.

  Complications include intravascular injection, dural puncture and technical difficulty due to anatomical variation (5%).
- Simple oral analgesia such as paracetamol is usually sufficient following the acute phase.

6. What methods of monitoring are available to detect air embolism? Briefly state the problems associated with each method.

- **Capnography** Air emboli are trapped in the pulmonary vessels causing a rapid rise in physiological dead space and an abrupt decrease in ET CO_2. Able to detect 1.5 ml/kg prior to cardiovascular collapse.
- **Awake patient** will complain of chest pain and dyspnoea preceding cardiovascular collapse.
- **Basic senses and a high index of suspicion.** At risk operations include neurosurgical and orthopaedic. Hissing may be heard over the surgical field. This is subjective and insensitive.
- **Heart sounds.** Millwheel murmur heard using a praecordial stethoscope. Insensitive needing 1.5–4.0 ml of air/kg by which time there may be cardiovascular collapse.
- **ECG.** Signs of right ventricular strain or arrhythmias. Non-specific.
- **CVP.** An abrupt rise due to outflow obstruction of the right heart. Again non-specific.

- **Transthoracic Doppler.** Placed in the 4th right interspace it can detect 0.5 ml of air by change in signal. However, oversensitivity (0.5 ml of air may be inconsequential), interference from diathermy and difficulty maintaining patient contact limit its use.
- **Transoesophageal echocardiography.** More sensitive than Doppler but will not differentiate between air, fat or blood microemboli.

7. What are the advantages and disadvantages of the interscalene versus the axillary approaches to the brachial plexus block?

Technical ease

- Interscalene has more difficult landmarks than the axillary approach, with its constant relationship to the axillary artery.
- Axillary approach allows easier placement of indwelling catheter for repeated injections.

Clinical application

- Interscalene reliably blocks structures innervated by C5–C7; the deep tissues of the shoulder, elbow joint and superficial areas of the radial aspect of the forearm. However, it inconsistently blocks the lower roots of the plexus.
- Axillary approach consistently blocks the medial aspects of arm, forearm and hand (median and ulnar nerves); however, radial and musculocutaneous nerves are blocked in only 75% cases and the circumflex nerve is unreliably blocked.

Complications

- Those of interscalene are numerous and may be serious compared with axillary block.

Interscalene

- Phrenic nerve block: 36% patients radiographically
- Recurrent laryngeal nerve block, hoarseness
- Horner's syndrome: 50% patients
- Vertebral artery injection, causing severe cerebral toxicity
- Epidural and subarachnoid injection.

Axillary

- Haematoma, especially if transarterial method is used
- Intravascular injection.

8. Write a letter to be carried by a patient who is thought to be susceptible to malignant hyperthermia.

To whom it may concern:
Re: AR Bloggs
DOB: ?/??/??

This patient developed masseter spasm following an appendicectomy and was subsequently investigated for malignant hyperthermia. A biopsy of vastus medialis showed contraction to both caffeine (2 mmol/l) and halothane (2%). This patient is therefore **malignant hyperthermia susceptible**.

If general anaesthesia is necessary, a volatile-free anaesthetic machine (produced by flushing a vaporiser-free machine with oxygen 8 l/min for 20 min) should be used together with a new ventilator and tubing.

Suxamethonium, all volatiles, amide local anaesthetics and sympathetic vasoconstrictors should all be avoided during anaesthesia. Monitoring should include temperature, capnography and oximetry. Dantrolene should be available within the operating theatre.

A national register of MH-susceptible individuals is kept in Leeds, from which further information may be obtained.

Yours sincerely

9. Outline the specific complications related to laparoscopic surgery.

Cardiovascular collapse

- Raised intra-abdominal pressure (IAP), reduced venous return and high systemic vascular resistance lead to low cardiac output. Aim to keep the IAP <15 mmHg and ensure normovolaemia.

Respiratory compromise

- Pneumoperitoneum splints the diaphragm, reduces FRC and compliance and therefore worsens ventilation/perfusion mismatch, resulting in hypoxaemia and hypercarbia. This is compounded by peritoneal absorption of carbon dioxide leading to acidosis and dysrhythmias.

Gas embolism

- Due to insertion of trochar into blood vessel. Carbon dioxide used as insufflating gas is highly soluble, to reduce this risk.

Visceral damage

- Due to limited view via the scope it may go unnoticed presenting as peritonitis at a later date.

Haemorrhage

- May be difficult to assess, especially if retroperitoneal.

Hypothermia

- Particularly a problem with long operations and use of cold insufflating gas.
- Venous stasis and thromboembolism.
- Due to high intra-abdominal pressures obstructing flow in the inguinal veins.

Escape of insufflating gas

- Pneumothorax or pneumoperitoneum may occur if the pleuroperitoneal canals are patent. Surgical emphysema and shoulder tip pain are common.

Ref: Kaufman L. *Anaesthesia Review*, 13th edn. 1996. London@ Churchill Livingstone.

10. What are the causes of hypoxaemia in the first 24 h following surgery? (60%) How do you reduce its occurrence? (40%)

Causes of hypoxaemia

- Hypoventilation due to airway obstruction, central depression from residual anaesthetic agents and opioids, obstructive sleep apnoea, pain or diaphragmatic splinting.
- Ventilation/perfusion mismatch and shunt. Due to atelectasis, mucus plugging, pulmonary oedema, aspiration, pulmonary embolus.
- Diffusion impairment due to pulmonary oedema or ARDS.
- Diffusion hypoxia; when a patient is emerging from anaesthesia with nitrous oxide, rapid outpouring of N_2O displaces alveolar oxygen resulting in hypoxia.
- Reduction in cardiac output or oxygen-carrying capacity.
- Increased oxygen consumption, shivering or systemic inflammatory response syndrome (SIRS).

Prevention

- Give supplemental oxygen to all those at risk of hypoventilation, for example all those receiving parenteral opioids.

- Give chest physiotherapy for at-risk groups such as smokers, those with chronic respiratory disease, the obese and all those having abdominal or thoracic surgery.
- Optimise pain relief for major intra-abdominal or thoracic operations in order to preserve respiratory function and aid physiotherapy.
- Administer 100% oxygen at the end of anaesthesia when using nitrous oxide.
- Optimise oxygen delivery, treat anaemia and improve cardiac output if necessary.
- Maintain body temperature and avoid shivering.
- Optimise ventilation/perfusion relationships using CPAP, non-invasive or invasive ventilation.

11. Outline the problems associated with anaesthetising a patient with sickle cell disease for an elective cholecystectomy.

- An inherited group of disorders characterised by variable amounts of haemoglobin S. Patients are usually SS but may be SC or S beta thal.
- Haemoglobin S in the deoxygenated form becomes insoluble, forming sickle-shaped red cells. A process promoted by hypoxia, acidosis, dehydration and low temperature.
- Chronic sickling leads to reduced microvascular blood flow (and end-organ damage) and chronic haemolytic anaemia (Hb 6–10 g/dl) with frequent gall stones.

Problems

Evaluation of pre-existing end-organ damage

- Cardiomegaly or cardiomyopathy. Raised cardiac output due to anaemia.
- Occult pulmonary infarction, possible pulmonary hypertension.
- Renal medullary infarction with impaired renal function and concentrating ability.

Prevention of peri-operative sickle crisis

- Consultation with a haematologist. Exchange transfusion over 6–8 weeks preoperatively may be indicated, aiming for Hb >8 g/dl and HbA >40%.
- Pre-, peri- and post-operative hypoxia, acidosis, hypothermia and dehydration are avoided.
- Sedative premedication is avoided. Intravenous hydration from the time of starvation.

- Preoxygenation with a smooth anaesthetic induction, intubation and moderate hyperventilation.
- Adequate warmed fluid replacement to maintain cardiac output and prevent vascular sludging.
- Careful intra-operative monitoring including pulse oximetry, urine output and temperature with use of active warming measures if necessary.
- Postoperative high dependency unit care to ensure adequate analgesia, avoidance of hypoxia, dehydration or hypotension.

Increased risk of infection

- Auto splenectomy places patients at increased risk, prophylactic antibiotics are advisable.

12. How would you preoperatively assess a patient due for a left pneumonectomy for a bronchogenic carcinoma?

General assessment

Preoperative assessment including history, examination and investigation.

Patients tend to be elderly, present or past smokers with concurrent cardio-respiratory disease.

Assessment of cardiorespiratory function

- Clinical examination to detect dyspnoea at rest or on exertion, sputum production and purulence, signs of right ventricular failure or bronchospasm.
- ECG to detect signs of right ventricular strain or ischaemic heart disease.
- CXR and ABGs to document baseline values.
- Full blood count and electrolytes.
- CT scan of the chest may indicate any tracheal deviation or large airway collapse.
- Lung function tests. These will also be useful in predicting the risk of pneumonectomy. Peak expiratory flow rate (PEFR) spirometry to produce FEV_1 and FVC and any response to bronchodilators.

Assessment of any paraneoplastic syndrome

- Bronchial carcinomas frequently produce hormone-like substances. Resulting biochemical abnormalities may need correction preoperatively.
- Hypercalcaemia from PTH-like substance.
- Inappropriate ADH.

- Cushing's syndrome.
- Eaton–Lambert syndrome: non-fatigable weakness of skeletal muscle.

Evaluation of the risk of pneumonectomy

- Left pneumonectomy comprises 40% of lung function. However, preoperative lung function may reflect a functional pneumonectomy if the lesion is occluding the main bronchus.
- No clear-cut criteria exist for selection of patients who will tolerate a pneumonectomy.

However, FEV_1 >0.8 l is needed for an adequate cough.

Patients with FEV_1 <1.0 l may have difficulty clearing secretions.

Maximal breathing capacity (MBC) <35 l/min correlates with poor outcome (MBC = PEFR ×0.25; or MBC = FEV_1 ×35).

Postoperative pulmonary hypertension is a significant cause of mortality. Efforts are now made to mimic the postoperative situation using pulmonary artery catheters. Mean pulmonary artery pressures > 40 mmHg are indicative of poor outcome.

Multiple Choice Question Paper 3 Answers

1 A trial has shown that a new cardiac output monitoring device has reduced mortality in surgery for fractured neck of femur from 10% to 8% Answers: A B C

From the available data for each 100 patients given the new device 8 died, compared to 10 in 100 control patients, a reduction of 20%. If there were only 50 patients per group then the number of patients who died were 4 and 5 respectively, rates likely by chance if there were no real differences between groups (the null hypothesis). If each group had 5000 patients the number of patients who died were 400 and 500 respectively, which is very unlikely by chance if there were no real differences between groups. If 100 patients received the new device 2 lives would be saved, so the number needed to treat is 50.

2 Pulse oximeters Answers: A B D

Pulse oximeters do not usually cause burns, but they can do in special circumstances such as in the MRI scanner or in patients receiving light-activated cytotoxics. Although they do not read in real time they are nevertheless much faster than transcutaneous oxygen electrodes. Pigmented skin does not affect the accuracy of pulse oximeters, but some nail varnishes do. In tricuspid regurgitation the device can pick up venous pulsations instead of arterial.

3 Measurement of oxygen in gases Answer: E

The concentration of oxygen in a mixture of gases may be measured by mass spectrometry or a paramagnetic analyser. The Clark electrode and the fuel cell can measure the oxygen tension in blood and in a mixture of gases, respectively.

The pulse oximeter measures the saturation of haemoglobin with oxygen.

The Severinghaus electrode measures the carbon dioxide tension in blood and the infrared analyser measures carbon dioxide tension in a mixture of gases.

The transcutaneous electrode measures the oxygen tension in blood in vivo.

4 Magnetic resonance scanning **Answers: B C D**

Pacemakers are a contraindication to a patient entering the MRI scanner. A quench is due to a sudden leak of helium or nitrogen and can result in sudden asphyxia. Monitoring may affect and be affected by MRI.

All ferromagnetic objects must be outside the 50-G field.

5 The gas laws **Answers: A C**

A is Boyle's law. P/T = constant is Charles's law. C is Henry's law. Graham actually found that larger molecules diffuse more slowly than smaller molecules. The universal gas constant is represented by the letter R (n is the number of moles of gas in $PV = nRT$).

6 Automated occlusive cuff blood pressure monitors **Answers: A B**

There is a little confusion in the textbooks on this subject. They measure systolic and MAP, and calculate diastolic pressure. The accuracy is usually good compared to invasive BP measurements, but is worse at extremes of pressure, tending to under read at high BP and over read at low BP. They require regular maintenance and calibration. The WHO recommends that an adult cuff is at least 14 cm wide.

7 Nitrous oxide can be measured by **Answers: A C D E**

Mass spectrometry, chromatography and Raman light scattering are techniques capable of measuring all gases. Nitrous oxide is one of the gases which absorb infrared. Oxygen is the only clinically useful gas that demonstrates the physical property of paramagnetism.

8 The 'train of four' measurement of neuromuscular blockade **Answers: A D E**

Serial reduction in twitch height occurs with non-depolarising muscle relaxants, there is no reduction with a depolarising block. Two detectable twitches equates to 80% of receptors blocked. It is painful in awake patients.

9 Concerning temperature **Answers: A B C D E**

0°C is 273 K. The saturated vapour pressure of water is 50 kPa at 80°C, and as liquids boil when the saturated vapour pressure equals atmospheric pressure water will boil at lower temperatures if the atmospheric pressure is reduced. Thermistors are semiconductors. Their resistance decreases in a non-linear way with increases in temperature.

10 In transthoracic echocardiography **Answers: A C E**

Normal aortic valves have an area of 2.5–3.5 cm^2. In moderate stenosis the valve area is 0.5–1.0 cm^2, in severe stenosis the aortic valve area is <0.5 cm^2. It is the technique of choice for diagnosing pericardial effusions. When combined with Doppler estimates of blood velocity, pressures in the pulmonary artery can be estimated.

11 Bronchial neoplasms **Answers: A C D**

Bronchial carcinomas may produce a variety of ectopic hormones such as ACTH, causing Cushing's syndrome with hypokalaemia, and parathormone causing hypercalcaemia. The syndrome of inappropriate production of antidiuretic hormone (SIADH) may occur. Hypercalcaemia can also occur if there are bony secondaries.

12 A laboratory report reading as follows **Answer: A**

SIADH leads to retention of water and both the serum sodium and potassium are reduced. Bowel obstruction with vomiting leads to hypokalaemia. In hepatic failure the urea is low as the liver fails to synthesise it. In renal failure the serum sodium is normal and there is no hypoglycaemia. Addison's disease fits the metabolic picture precisely.

Lack of cortisol leads to loss of sodium chloride and retention of potassium, as well as hypoglycaemia. The urea is elevated and there is a metabolic acidosis.

13 Head injury **Answers: A C D**

An extradural haematoma following a head injury is due to bleeding from the middle meningeal artery. It requires surgical evacuation. Persistent CSF rhinorrhoea and a depressed skull fracture will also require surgery, but a linear fracture does not. Convulsions require treatment with anticonvulsants but do not necessarily indicate that the patient requires surgery.

14 Serum creatine phosphokinase **Answers: A E**

The enzyme creatine kinase (CK) has three iso-enzymes:
(1) CK-BB found in brain tissue
(2) CK-MM found in muscle tissue
(3) CK-MB found in myocardial tissue

An elevated creatine kinase can be seen 24 h after a myocardial infarct, in Duchenne muscular dystrophy and in hypothyroidism.

Osteomalacia leads to an increase in the enzyme alkaline phosphatase, which can be produced by osteoblasts or hepatocytes; hence it is elevated in liver disease as well.

15 Carcinoma of the bronchus **Answers: A C D E**

Carcinoma of the bronchus is associated with a number of non-metastatic extrathoracic complications. These include the Eaton–Lambert myasthenic syndrome, peripheral neuropathy, cerebellar degeneration and dementia. The tumour can cause superior vena caval obstruction and may, rarely, cause a lymphocytic meningitis.

16 Hyperkalaemia **Answers: A C**

Hyperkalaemia leads to a prolonged PR interval, flattened P waves, widened QRS complexes and tall peaked T waves. Hypokalaemia is associated with U waves; delta waves are seen in the Wolf–Parkinson–White syndrome.

17 Unconjugated bilirubin **Answers: D E**

Bilirubin is rendered water soluble by conjugation with glucuronide by the hepatocytes. Unconjugated bilirubin is bound to albumin but readily crosses the neonatal blood–brain barrier and can cause kernicterus.

Phenobarbitone induces liver microsomal enzymes and enhances the conjugation process.

18 Addison's disease **Answer: C**

Addison's disease is primary adrenocortical insufficiency (ACTH is high already). Lack of aldosterone and cortisol leads to loss of sodium and water and hence low blood pressure (particularly postural hypotension). There is hyperkalaemia, a mild metabolic acidosis and an inability to excrete a water load. It is treated with hydrocortisone and fludrocortisone.

19 Ritodrine **Answer: C**

Ritodrine is an agonist at beta-2 adrenoreceptors. It is used specifically to arrest premature labour. Like salbutamol, another beta-2 agonist, it produces tachycardia, peripheral vasodilatation and hypotension. Other side-effects include hypokalaemia and pulmonary oedema.

20 Ionised calcium **Answers: A B C D E**

The total blood calcium consists of ionised (free) calcium and protein-bound calcium. The ionised calcium is affected by pH and the serum albumin. The binding of calcium to albumin is pH dependent such that a rise in pH (alkalosis) leads to a reduction in the ionised fraction. As calcium is bound to albumin the serum calcium has to be adjusted by adding 0.2 mmol/l for every 10 g that the albumin is below 45 g/l.

21 Drug induced hyperglycaemia **Answers: A C E**

The thiazides may cause hyperglycaemia. All steroids including the OCP can impair glucose tolerance. Although the beta blockers can mask the autonomic response to hypoglycaemia they do not impair glucose tolerance.

22 Persistent vomiting **Answers: B D E**

Persistent vomiting leads to dehydration and other metabolic problems that must be corrected prior to surgery. In pyloric stenosis there is obstruction to gastric outlet and so the vomitus will be free of bile. Duodenal atresia is associated with Down's syndrome.

23 Transplantation of the ureter in the colon **Answers: B D**

Transplantation of the ureter in the colon is the textbook example of a condition causing a hyperchloraemic acidosis. There is reabsorption of urinary urea by the colonic mucosa causing a rise in blood urea. There is hypokalaemia caused by the kidneys' attempts to retain bicarbonate in exchange for hydrogen and potassium ions.

24 Dopamine **Answers: A C D**

Dopamine is a naturally occurring sympathetic amine; the endogenous precursor of noradrenaline. At low doses (2–4 mg/kg per min) dopamine stimulates dopamine 1 and 2 receptors, increasing renal blood flow, glomerular filtration rate and sodium excretion. Between 3 and 10 μg/kg per min dopamine stimulates beta-1 receptors causing positive inotropy and chronotropy. At doses above 10 mg/kg per min dopamine activates alpha receptors causing systemic vasoconstriction.

There is currently much debate about the rationale for using low-dose dopamine therapy in acute renal failure. Dopamine must be administered via a central line. It does not cross the blood–brain barrier.

Ref: McCrory C and Cunningham A J. Low-dose dopamine: will there ever be a scientific rationale? *Br J Anaesth* 1997; **78**: 350–351.

25 Clonidine — Answers: A B C D

Clonidine is a mixed alpha-2 and alpha-1 adrenergic agonist (alpha-2: alpha-1 activity 200:1). It may be given orally, intravenously or epidurally. It produces hypotension by reducing central sympathetic outflow. The resulting unopposed parasympathetic vagal tone causes bradycardia. It is also an antisialogue, anxiolytic and sedative. Like the other alpha-2 agonists dexmedetomidine and medetomidine it reduces the minimum alveolar concentration of volatile agents by up to 50%. Dexmedetomidine is used in veterinary anaesthetics as an induction agent and for maintenance of anaesthesia. It is even more selective for alpha-2 receptors than clonidine.

26 Infantile pyloric stenosis — Answer: A

Infantile pyloric stenosis causes projectile vomiting of gastric contents. The metabolic consequences are due to loss of HCl from the stomach; thus there is a metabolic alkalosis and hypochloraemia. The renal response to the resulting dehydration is to retain sodium and water in preference to correcting the alkalosis. Thus there is paradoxical aciduria and renal loss of potassium causing hypokalaemia. This is a medical, but not a surgical, emergency. The priority is to correct the dehydration and acid–base disturbance prior to surgery.

27 Stridor — Answers: A B C D

Stridor is caused by glottic obstruction, due to oedema or a foreign body, and may be seen in croup, epiglottitis or tonsillitis. Bronchiolitis is caused by viral inflammation of the lower respiratory tract.

28 Neonatal physiology **Answers: A B D**

In the neonate the stroke volume is relatively fixed and cardiac output increases are rate dependent. The liver is immature at birth and levels of vitamin-K-dependent clotting factors are low. The oxygen consumption of the neonate is approximately twice that of an adult. Circulating blood volume of the neonate is about 80–100 ml/kg.

29 Acute epiglottitis **Answer: C**

Acute epiglottitis is a bacterial infection most often caused by *Haemophilus influenzae* type B. After the introduction of the HIB vaccine the incidence initially fell, but is now beginning to rise again. While most cases occur in children it may occur in adults. Ampicillin or chloramphenicol are the antibiotics most often used. Intravenous access should wait until after a gentle inhalational induction; trying to secure venous access early may lead to total airway obstruction. Once the pyrexia has settled and there is an audible leak around the endotracheal tube, extubation is possible; usually after 24–48 h.

30 Obstructive sleep apnoea **Answers: B C D**

There is intermittent upper airways obstruction. May be precipitated or exacerbated by alcohol or sedatives (so premedication should be avoided). If severe it can progress to cor pulmonale. Treatment includes: weight loss; avoidance of precipitants; nasal CPAP; uvulopharyngopalatoplasty; and tracheostomy if necessary. These patients have a high perioperative risk, and should usually go to HDU postoperatively.

31 Cervical cord injury **Answers: A B C D**

The combination of hypotension and bradycardia suggests neurogenic shock and is due to loss of sympathetic vasomotor tone and the cardio-accelerator fibres. Although ultimately there will be signs of spasticity, due to upper motor neurone damage, initially there is spinal shock. Spinal shock is manifest, as is areflexic flaccidity of the limbs.

Damage to the phrenic nerve (C3, 4, 5) occurs with high cervical cord injuries and leads to paralysis of the diaphragm. Lower lesions may only affect the intercostal muscles with less respiratory impairment.

32 Intra-aortic balloon **Answers: D E**

The intra-aortic balloon pump (IABP) is inserted via the femoral artery and positioned in the descending aorta, just distal to the left subclavian artery. Inflation is synchronised to the patient's ECG. It is inflated with 50 ml of helium or carbon dioxide at the onset of diastole. This results in displacement of blood into the proximal and distal aorta, increasing aortic diastolic pressure. This in turn leads to improved coronary artery perfusion and increased myocardial oxygen delivery. It is deflated just prior to systole so decreasing left ventricular afterload, left ventricular work and myocardial oxygen requirements.

33 Shock following trauma **Answer: B**

Neurogenic shock implies a significant head injury; there is nothing in the history to suggest this. A ruptured urethra would not cause shock. Fat embolism usually occurs later than 1 h after the accident and causes hypoxia and confusion. Shock is not a major feature. Blood loss is the likeliest explanation for the clinical findings.

34 Increasing intracranial pressure **Answers: A B E**

Increasing intracranial pressure may lead to headache and vomiting, neurological signs (eg VIth nerve palsy), seizures and a decline in the Glasgow coma score. Classically there is hypertension with reflex bradycardia, the Cushing response, although in practice this is probably just one end of a spectrum of general cardiovascular instability because tachycardias may also occur. The pupils are dilated and respiratory depression leads to an increase in P_aCO_2.

35 Tension pneumothorax **Answers: C D**

The clinical findings are those of a tension pneumothorax, which is a medical emergency. The patient requires oxygen and immediate needling of the right side of the chest. Once stabilised a chest drain with underwater seal can be inserted until the right lung has completely re-expanded.

36 Chronic respiratory acidosis **Answer: B**

Chronic respiratory acidosis is due to carbon dioxide retention, as occurs in chronic bronchitis. To restore pH towards normal the kidneys retain bicarbonate ions and excrete hydrogen ions.

37 Paracetamol poisoning **Answers: D E**

It is salicylate poisoning that is associated with an early metabolic acidosis and hyperventilation. The main danger of paracetamol poisoning is liver damage. Normally 90% of paracetamol is conjugated by the liver with glucuronide or sulphate and excreted by the kidneys. A small amount is converted to a toxic metabolite which is normally then conjugated with glutathione and excreted by the kidneys. In overdose the glutathione is exhausted leaving the toxic metabolite free to cause centrilobular necrosis of the liver. Either oral methionine or intravenous *N*-acetylcysteine can be used as treatment up to 24 h after the overdose to prevent the hepatic damage by the toxic metabolite. They act by replenishing the exhausted glutathione stores and mopping up the reactive metabolite.

38 Oliguria **Answers: B E**

Oliguria is the excretion of a urine volume too low for renal homeostatic mechanisms to maintain normal blood concentrations of waste products.

The result is a rise in the plasma concentrations of urea, creatinine and potassium. In acute tubular necrosis (ATN) small amounts of poor quality urine are produced. Since the tubules fail to reabsorb sodium adequately it is found in high concentrations in the urine. The urine itself has a low osmolality and there is a failure to excrete urea, with a low urinary urea. The CVP rises as the kidneys fail to excrete water; ultimately this may lead to pulmonary oedema.

By comparison oliguria due to pre-renal failure is a physiological response to poor renal perfusion and leads to the production of small amounts of concentrated urine. As the kidneys are actually functioning normally the response is to conserve sodium, so the urinary sodium is low, while urea is appropriately excreted and the urinary urea is high.

Most cases of pre-renal failure are due to hypovolaemia from dehydration or haemorrhage. Thus the CVP is low and the treatment is to give fluids and/or blood to expand the vascular volume and return renal perfusion to normal. This is clearly not appropriate management for ATN, and is why it is important to differentiate correctly between the two causes of oliguria.

39 Cardiac arrest **Answers: A C D E**

The chances of survival following cardiac arrest when the rhythm is VF decline exponentially with the time taken to defibrillation. If a VF arrest is witnessed, for example in a patient in CCU with ECG monitoring attached, then often a simple pre-cordial thump will restore sinus rhythm.

Calcium is only indicated in cases of electro-mechanical dissociation (or PEA – pulseless electrical activity as it is now known) associated with hypocalcaemia or hyperkalaemia or the patient is on a calcium channel blocker. An 8.4% sodium bicarbonate solution is hyperosmolar. Its use is controversial as it may actually worsen intracellular acidosis. The latest ERC recommendations are that bicarbonate should only be used if resuscitation is prolonged and where blood gases show an acidosis in the context of normocapnoea. There is some evidence to show that cooling the patient for 24 h may offer some benefits in terms of neurological outcome.

40 Tetanus **Answers: A B C D**

Tetanus results from the actions of the exotoxin (tetanospasmin) of the bacillus *Clostridium tetani*. Tetanospasmin leads to generalised muscle rigidity and sympathetic overactivity. There may be respiratory compromise requiring ventilation. Human antitetanus antitoxin will neutralise exotoxin not yet fixed in the CNS. Active immunisation with tetanus toxoid prevents the disease, but boosters are required every 10 years or on injury if the last booster was more than 5 years previously.

The incubation period is 2–45 days.

41 Central venous pressure **Answers: A B C D**

The central venous pressure is a measure of right heart filling pressure (preload).The most accurate readings are obtained if the catheter tip lies in the lower superior vena cava or the right atrium. The classical a, c and v waves are transmitted from the right atrium to the internal jugular vein but are not seen in the axillary vein. With IPPV the normal physiological drop in CVP with inspiration is reversed as the intrathoracic pressure rises and blood is pushed out of the thoracic cavity.

42 Cardioversion **Answers: B E**

DC is used rather than AC for cardioversion. Sedation may be adequate rather than general anaesthesia. The shock should be at the start of the QRS complex. R on T may occur if the shock is not synchronised, resulting in VF. For elective cardioversion preoperative preparation includes anticoagulation and correction of electrolytes (K^+ and Mg^{2+}).

43 Ecstasy (MDMA) **Answers: A B C E**

It is estimated that Ecstasy or MDMA (3,4-methylenedioxymethamphetamine) may lead to about 50 deaths annually in the UK. Like other amphetamines its injection causes sympathetic stimulation with tachycardia, hypertension, myriasis and sweating. With profound sympathetic overactivity there may be hyperpyrexia, rhabdomyolysis, myoglobinuria and acute renal failure with DIC, convulsions, hyperkalaemia and metabolic acidosis; coma and death may supervene.

In some deaths from MDMA water intoxication has caused death from acute cerebral oedema. There are many similarities with malignant hyperpyrexia and dantrolene is now used to treat MDMA intoxication.

Parkinsonism can result from ingestion of the 'designer drug' MPTP, which has a high degree of cytotoxicity for the substantia nigra.

44 Hypothermia **Answers: B D**

Hypothermia may occur in the elderly especially in winter if they collapse and are not discovered for some time. It may occur following a stroke, immersion in cold water, hypothyroidism, alcohol and drug intoxication. Myocardial depression, bradycardia with a J wave on the ECG, and arrhythmias can occur below 28°C. There is usually a metabolic acidosis, and complications such as acute pancreatitis, hyperglycaemia, thrombocytopenia and DIC may occur.

45 Carbon monoxide poisoning **Answers: B C D**

Carbon monoxide (CO) has an affinity for haemoglobin of 250 times that of oxygen. The result is reduced oxygen carriage by haemoglobin and reduced oxygen delivery to the tissues. There is left shift of the oxyhaemoglobin dissociation curve. In addition there is histotoxic hypoxia as CO binds to and inhibits the enzymes of cellular respiration.

The severity of the situation may be masked as the pulse oximeter overestimates the oxygen saturation, and the arterial oxygen tension is normal. Clinically CO poisoning produces tachycardia, decreased level of consciousness, convulsions and coma. There is often a metabolic (lactic) acidosis and hypokalaemia. The carboxyhaemoglobin (COHb) level must be measured to guide treatment. All patients should receive 100% oxygen. At a COHb level of >40% hyperbaric oxygen therapy (HBO) should be considered. Since: $C_aO_2 = Hb \times 1.34 + (P_aO_2 \times 0.03)$ where C_aO_2 is oxygen content, and $DO_2 = CaO_2 \times CO$ DO_2 is oxygen delivery and CO is cardiac output. With HBO therapy, at 300 kPa, the P_aO_2 is sufficient, assuming a normal cardiac output, to meet average tissue oxygen requirements.

46 Intubation and ventilation of an elderly man **Answers: A B C D E**

This man requires intubation and ventilation in view of his hypoxia and GCS of 6. The blood gases reveal a metabolic acidosis with an increased anion gap.

The anion gap formula is Na + K – HCO_3 + Cl. The normal range is 9–14 mmol/l.
Causes of a metabolic acidosis with a raised anion gap include:
Lactic acidosis
Ketoacidosis
Renal failure
Salicylate and methanol poisoning
Rhabdomyolysis.

The glucose of 10 mmol/l does not rule out the diagnosis of diabetic keto-acidosis – he may have had a dose of insulin before collapsing.

47 Overdose of cocaine **Answers: A B C**

The manifestations of cocaine overdose include agitated delirium, seizures, hyperthermia with rhabdomyolysis, refractory chest pain and hypertension. The mainstay of therapy is sedation with benzodiazepines and cooling. Phenothiazines are contraindicated as they may precipitate dystonic reactions, impair heat dissipation and lower the seizure threshold. α adrenergic antagonists are used to treat coronary vasospasm and refractory hypertension.

48 In acute pancreatitis **Answers: C E**

Ninety percent of cases of pancreatitis are oedematous interstitial which carries a better prognosis than necrotising pancreatitis. In 30%–40% of cases overlying gas renders the pancreas difficult to visualise by ultrasound, thus contrast-enhanced CT is the imaging method of choice. Necrotising pancreatitis, characterised by high levels of LDH and CRP, commonly progresses to MODS and may be treated by surgical resection.

49 Concerning rhabdomyolysis **Answer: C**

Calcium accumulates in damaged muscle leading to hypocalcaemia in early rhabdomyolysis. Myoglobinaemia as well as acidosis causes direct renal vasoconstriction. Alkalinisation increases the solubility of the Tamm Horsfall protein–myoglobin complex and is used in treatment. Myoglobin is rapidly metabolised by the liver and its absence does not exclude the diagnosis. The prognosis is excellent.

50 Concerning electrocution **Answers: B D**

Ventricular fibrillation is the commonest presenting rhythm following an AC shock. The current follows the path of least resistance, often along neurovascular bundles thus transthoracic current is more likely to traverse the myocardium. Creatine kinase is also liberated from damaged muscle.

51 Malignant hyperpyrexia **Answers: A C**

The history points to a diagnosis of malignant hyperpyrexia as a possible cause of death in the patient's brother. The serum creatine phosphokinase is a useful marker for this condition but lacks both specificity and sensitivity.

A muscle biopsy is required so that the in vitro contracture tests can be performed. This involves exposing muscle to halothane and caffeine.

The fluoride number and plasma cholinesterase level are tests for the presence of atypical plasma cholinesterase, so-called scolene apnoea, also known as suxamethonium apnoea or pseudo choline esterase deficiency.

52 Oliguria **Answers: All false**

The preoperative blood urea of 10 mmol/l suggests existing renal disease. Postoperatively the patient's urea rises further and small amounts of poor quality urine are produced. The normal response to stress involves release of ADH and aldosterone leading to retention of sodium and water.

53 Extracellular depletion of body fluids **Answers: A B C D E**

In response to acute extracellular depletion of body fluids the kidneys produce renin and the pituitary produces ADH. There is a rise in blood urea and haemoconcentration. Renin leads to increased aldosterone release from the adrenal cortex which in turn leads to retention of sodium. The

ADH leads to water retention. The result is the production of small amounts of concentrated urine.

54 TUR syndrome **Answers: A C**

The TUR syndrome results from the absorption of large amounts of irrigating fluid into the vascular space. The biochemical effects are due to haemodilution and include hyponatraemia, hypokalaemia and hypocalcaemia. Irrigating fluid is isotonic and so does not cause haemolysis.

55 Right main bronchus **Answers: A C**

The right main bronchus, after 2.5 cm, gives off the right upper lobe bronchus, which in turn trifurcates to give the apical, anterior and posterior segments. The right main bronchus continues a further 2 cm before giving off the middle lobe bronchus, which in turn bifurcates into the lateral and medial segments of the right middle lobe. The right main bronchus, at 4.5 cm, is slightly shorter than the left which is 5 cm in length. The right main bronchus lies superior and posterior to the right pulmonary artery and inferior to the azygous vein.

56 Postoperative thyrotoxic crisis **Answers: A D**

To control the tachycardia and agitation of postoperative thyrotoxic crisis diazepam and propranolol should be given at once. Carbimazole will not work immediately and should be given once the initial situation is controlled.

57 Metabolic changes after partial gastrectomy **Answers: B D E**

After major surgery the body produces increased amounts of renin, ADH and cortisol leading to hyperglycaemia and renal retention of sodium and water and excretion of potassium. The patient is in a catabolic state and there is increased excretion of nitrogen and increased consumption of oxygen. Muscle and adipose tissue are broken down to supply energy leading to an increased level of circulating free fatty acids.

It is thought that many of these metabolic responses are mediated by cytokines, especially interleukin-1, interleukin-6 and tumour necrosis factor-alpha. The rise in IL-6 is a good measure of the degree of tissue injury, and there is evidence that anaesthesia can attenuate the rise in IL-6.

Ref: Masterson G R and Hunter J M. Does anaesthesia have long-term consequences? *Br J Anaesth* 1996; **77:** 569–570.

58 Osseous metastases due to prostate cancer **Answers: A C E**

The pain from bony metastases due to prostate cancer can be relieved by radiotherapy, orchiectomy or diethylstilbestrol. Opioids and NSAIDs may also be of benefit.

59 Carotid sheath **Answers: A B C**

The carotid sheath contains the carotid artery, internal jugular vein and the vagus nerve.

60 One-lung anaesthesia and the shunt equation **Answers: A D**

One of the problems with this sort of question is that what you observe thoracic anaesthetists doing does not always follow what would be predicted by the theory.

In this question the patient would be in the lateral position with the upper lung collapsed and the lower (dependent) lung being ventilated. There will be true shunt – some of the cardiac output still passing through the upper, unventilated lung. This will result in hypoxia that, according to the shunt equation, cannot be improved by increasing the F_iO_2. PEEP may be predicted to exacerbate hypoxia by diverting more of the cardiac output to the unventilated lung. Reducing the shunt fraction will improve oxygenation and this can be achieved physiologically by hypoxic pulmonary vasoconstriction or surgically by clamping the upper pulmonary artery. CPAP to the collapsed lung may reduce the shunt fraction, counteract the effect of PEEP to the dependent lung, and may enable blood passing through the upper lung to be oxygenated.

In practice if hypoxia is a problem anaesthetists tend to increase the F_iO_2, try dependent PEEP and try upper lung CPAP before moving on to reventilating the collapsed lung and asking the surgeon to ligate the upper artery.

61 Hypoxic mixture **Answers: B D E**

Acute hypoxia leads to central cyanosis, a reduced mixed venous oxygen content, as the tissues extract more oxygen to prevent tissue hypoxia and tachypnoea. The alveolar gas equation can be used to estimate the alveolar (and therefore the arterial) partial pressure of oxygen. The partial pressure of inspired oxygen is given by $F_iO_2 \times (P_B - P_AH_2O)$, in this case $0.1 \times (100-6.3) = 9.37$. The PO_2 is then $9.37 - P_ACO_2/R$. Taking R to be 0.8 the P_AO_2 can be calculated for various values of P_ACO_2. If the minute ventilation is normal the P_ACO_2 is about 5 kPa, therefore the P_AO_2 will be about 3.4 kPa. If the PCO_2 is 1.5, the P_AO_2 will be 7.5. If the PCO_2 is 6.5 the P_AO_2 will be 1 kPa.

62 Colloids **Answers: A B D E**

The colloids are plasma expanders. The four main types are given below.

(a) Gelatins (eg Haemaccel®, Gelofusine®)
They have a mol. wt. of 30 000–35 000 and an oncotic pressure similar to plasma. They do not cause renal failure or impair blood cross matching, but can cause allergic reactions. Haemaccel® contains calcium and will cause citrated blood to clot if it comes into contact.

(b) Dextrans (eg dextran 70)
The dextrans may cause renal failure, impair grouping and cross matching of blood and impair haemostasis by reducing factor 8 concentration and platelet adhesiveness.

(c) Starches (eg Hetastarch®)
Hetastarch® contains very large molecules of mol. wt. up to 450 000. Thus the plasma expansion is slightly greater than the volume of starch infused, and lasts in excess of 24 h. The starches can impair renal function and impair haemostasis, by prolongation of the APTT, PT and bleeding time. They cause reduced levels of factor 8 and von Willebrand's factor.
They are associated with a syndrome of intractable pruritus.
Ref: Warren B B and Durieux M E. Hydroxyethyl starch: safe or not? *Anesthesia Analgesia* 1997; **84**: 206–212.
Ref: Cone A. The use of colloids in clinical practice. *Br J Hosp Med* 1995; **54**: 155–159.

(d) Human albumin
4.5% human albumin has a very similar oncotic pressure to plasma, as the normal plasma albumin is about 45 g/l.
Ref: Soni N. Wonderful colloid? *Br Med J* 1995; **310**: 887–888.

63 Drugs precipitating bronchospasm **Answers: A B C**

Aspirin and the NSAIDs may produce bronchospasm. Morphine may cause histamine release and therefore produce bronchospasm. Labetalol, like all beta blockers, can cause bronchoconstriction. All the volatile agents are bronchodilators, as is ketamine.

64 Porphyric crisis **Answers: A B E**

The signs of a porphyric crisis include tachycardia, pyrexia, psychosis and the passing of urine which darkens on standing. Renal colic is not a symptom of porphyric crises but abdominal pain can occur.

65 Isoflurane **Answers: A C D E**

Isoflurane will absorb ultraviolet and infra-red radiation and will cause a change in the elasticity of silicone rubber. Isoflurane concentration can also be determined by a refractometer. Isoflurane has a mol. wt. of 184.5 daltons, and is therefore more dense than nitrous oxide (44 daltons).

Ref: Craft T M and Upton P M. *Key topics in anaesthesia*, 2nd edn. Oxford: Bios, pp 126–128.

66 Intraocular pressure (IOP) **Answers: A E**

Intraocular pressure (IOP) is raised by hypoxia, hypercarbia, hypertension and elevated venous pressure. Acetazolamide acts by inhibiting the enzyme carbonic anhydrase. The result is a reduced production of aqueous humour and a consequent reduction in intraocular pressure. Atropine, by causing mydriasis, improves aqueous drainage.

While all the volatile agents and both propofol and thiopentone reduce IOP, suxamethonium causes an increase in IOP.

67 Perioperative hyperkalaemia **Answers: A B E**

Suxamethonium normally leads to an increase in serum potassium of 0.5–1.0 mmol/l. Certain patients can develop greater rises in potassium, predisposing to malignant ventricular arrhythmias. Rhabdomyolysis from trauma produces hyperkalaemia. Blood contains a higher potassium than plasma; transfusion can cause hyperkalaemia. Intravenous bicarbonate and calcium gluconate are used to treat hyperkalaemia.

68 Nimodipine **Answers: A C D**

Nimodipine is a calcium-channel-blocking drug. It acts preferentially on cerebral arteries and is used specifically to prevent vasospasm and ischaemia following subarachnoid haemorrhage. Like all calcium antagonists it is a hypotensive agent. While diltiazem and verapamil enhance the effect of theophyllines, nimodipine has no effect.

69 Coeliac plexus block **Answers: A B C D E**

Coeliac plexus block is used to manage pain in conditions such as pancreatic cancer and chronic pancreatitis. Side-effects of the block include orthostatic hypotension, impotence and constriction of the sphincter of Oddi.

70 Reactions to intravenous dextrans **Answers: A B C D**

Dextran is a high molecular weight polysaccharide, Dextran having a molecular weight of 40 000. Dextran 40 causes clotting deficits, and it is used for this property in vascular and microvascular surgery. The incidence of allergic reactions to the dextrans is less than to most of the colloids, except for human albumin. The incidence of anaphylactoid reactions is <0.1%. Reactions can be reduced by pre-treatment with small haptan molecules, and Dextran 1 is licensed for this indication. This may explain why test doses or slow administration reduces reactions.

71 The following are absorbed transdermally **Answers: B D**

Hyoscine is marketed as a patch for motion sickness. Fentanyl is also available in a transdermal preparation for the treatment of malignant pain.

72 Propofol **Answers: B D**

Propofol is presented in a white aqueous emulsion containing 10% soyabean oil (intralipid), 1.2% purified egg phosphatide and 2.25% glycerol. It causes a drop in blood pressure of 15%–25%, due to a reduction in cardiac output and peripheral vasodilatation. There is usually a reflex tachycardia. Propofol usually causes apnoea after induction and decreases the ventilatory response to hypercarbia. It reduces intraocular pressure and, bizarre though it sounds, may cause green urine.

73 Bupivacaine **Answers: A B D E**

Bupivacaine is an amide local anaesthetic. It is highly protein bound. All the local anaesthetic agents are safe in malignant hyperpyrexia. The main disadvantage of the agent is its cardiotoxicity, especially in pregnant women. There have been reports of it leading to refractory ventricular fibrillation in parturients and when used for intravenous regional anaesthesia (IVRA).

74 Premature neonates **Answers: A B D E**

Premature neonates are more likely than term babies to suffer from hypothermia, hypocalcaemia and hypoglycaemia. They are often mildly jaundiced and are sensitive to the effects of the non-depolarising muscle relaxants.

75 Ventricular ectopics **Answers: A C**

Lignocaine is the treatment of choice for ventricular ectopic beats during anaesthesia. Ischaemia, hypercarbia, electrolyte imbalance and a high level of circulating catecholamines predispose to the problem. The beta-adrenoceptor blocking drugs may also prevent ventricular ectopics.

Carotid sinus pressure and verapamil may be used in supraventricular tachycardia, although adenosine is now first-line therapy. Digoxin increases ventricular excitability and is not a treatment for ventricular ectopics. Its use is in atrial fibrillation, especially if associated heart failure is present.

76 Acid aspiration **Answers: A B D**

Treatment of acid aspiration may involve bronchoscopy, bronchial lavage and ventilatory support. Steroids used to be thought to be of benefit. Antibiotics are usually not started unless there is evidence of infection. Diuretics are not relevant.

77 Oxytocin **Answers: A C**

Oxytocin (Syntocinon®) and ergometrine are used to induce or augment labour and to minimise blood loss from the placental site. Oxytocin is produced endogenously in the posterior pituitary. It has actions similar to those of the other posterior pituitary hormone, ADH. Thus it causes fluid retention, which can be severe enough to lead to water intoxication and convulsions when used as an infusion for prolonged periods. It causes peripheral vasodilatation with hypotension and reflex tachycardia. Oxytocin is very short acting.

Ergometrine has a faster onset of action, and its effects last up to several hours. It is a vasoconstrictor and causes hypertension and a high incidence of nausea and vomiting.

78 Agents to relax the uterus **Answers: A D E**

Thiopentone, halothane and the other volatile agents will all relax the uterus. Suxamethonium and the non-depolarising muscle relaxants act at the neuromuscular junction of striated muscle; they have no effect on the smooth muscle of the uterus. Ritodrine and salbutamol are beta 2 adrenergic receptor agonists and can be used to relax the uterus.

79 Cardiovascular changes in pregnancy **Answers: A C D**

The cardiovascular changes in pregnancy include an increase in heart rate and stroke volume and a fall in systemic vascular resistance. The result is that there is a fall in diastolic and mean blood pressure. Although total red cell mass increases there is a greater increase in plasma volume and hence a dilutional anaemia.

80 Anaphylactic reactions **Answers: B D E**

Anaphylactic reactions are type 1 hypersensitivity reactions, mediated by specific IgE antibodies. In a previously sensitised individual antigen and antibody bind to, and then lead to the degranulation of, mast cells and basophils. Release of histamine, serotonin and other cytokines leads to the clinical manifestations of urticaria, hypotension and bronchospasm. Anaphylactoid reactions are also the result of mast cell degranulation, but this is mediated directly by the drug, without involvement of IgE.

The most commonly implicated anaesthetic drugs include suxamethonium and some non-depolarising muscle relaxants, opioids, penicillins and NSAIDs. The colloids and latex rubber are important aetiologically to anaesthetists. Treatment must include adrenaline as a first-line drug. Its alpha agonist effect reverses vasodilatation and its beta agonist effect reverses bronchoconstriction and increases the force of myocardial contraction. Oxygen and plasma volume expansion are required.

Antihistamines and corticosteroids are useful second-line drugs.

Salbutamol, aminophylline, isoflurane and ketamine may be used for refractory bronchospasm.

When investigating a reaction the serum mast cell tryptase is a sensitive and specific test for confirming that mast cell degranulation has occurred. Referral of the patient to an immunologist allows identification of the allergen by demonstrating specific IgE antibodies by either skinprick test or radio-allergosorbent test (RAST).

A CSM Yellow Card should be filled in and the patient's GP informed.

The patient should be fully informed and encouraged to carry an anaesthetic hazard card or wear a Medic-alert bracelet.

Ref: The Association of Anaesthetists of Great Britain and Ireland. *Suspected anaphylactic reactions associated with anaesthesia*, 2nd edn. 1995. London: The Association of Anaesthetists of Great Britain and Ireland.

81 Cardiopulmonary bypass **Answer: D**

Venous drainage is under gravity via the right atrium or superior and inferior vena cava. Blood is oxygenated by diffusion through membrane oxygenators. Bubble oxygenators force tiny bubbles of gas into the blood. Defoaming removes bubbles, detergent should never be mixed with blood. The pump is primed with crystalloid or colloid or sometimes blood. The prime volume is 1.5–2.5 l.

82 The maxillary nerve **Answers: A E**

The maxillary nerve (V^2) supplies sensation to the temple, cheek, nose, palate and upper teeth. From its origin at the trigeminal (Gasserian) ganglion it passes through the foramen rotundum to the pterygopalatine fossa. The posterior superior alveolar branch supplies sensation to the upper molar teeth. It may be blocked in the pterygopalatine fossa via an intra oral route, or by an extra oral route.

Although this area of anatomy seems small print, it is important: dental surgeons routinely block branches of the nerve; it can be affected by trigeminal neuralgia; and it regularly features in the Final FRCA basic sciences viva.

83 Anaesthetic management of a woman who is 8 weeks pregnant **Answers: B D**

In the first trimester the extra risks of anaesthesia are teratogenicity and spontaneous abortion. Diazepam has been implicated as being associated with cleft palate, and nitrous oxide is best avoided because of its effect on methionine synthesis (and therefore DNA). Hypoxia is teratogenic, maternal hyperoxia causes no problems. Safe drugs include thiopentone, propofol, fentanyl, morphine (although a problem if used chronically), volatiles, muscle relaxants, lignocaine and bupivacaine, The use of NSAIDs is controversial, but they are usually avoided because of the theoretical risk of causing closure of the ductus arteriosus.

A rapid sequence induction is only indicated routinely from the start of the second trimester. Regional techniques are often preferable where possible, providing anaesthesia, prolonged analgesia and avoidance of polypharmacy.

84 Repair of ruptured abdominal aortic aneurysm — Answers: all false

Emergency repair of ruptured aortic aneurysm has a mortality of >50%. A femoral arterial line has nothing to record when the cross-clamp is placed, and so a radial or brachial line is preferred. Renal dysfunction is common, even for elective repair with a cross-clamp below the level of the renal arteries. Paraplegia commonly is the result of thrombosis of the anterior spinal artery. Epidural analgesia, although potentially useful, is rarely done because of concerns about coagulopathy.

85 Anaesthetic management of post-tonsillectomy haemorrhage — Answers: D E

Haemorrhage post-tonsillectomy is an emergency. Large volumes of blood may be swallowed, making estimation of blood loss difficult and causing a 'full stomach'. The initial management is ABC and the blood volume should be restored before re-anaesthetising. NSAIDs have been implicated in the aetiology of early haemorrhage, and their use is controversial, but should definitely be avoided if there is rebleeding. It is occasionally the presenting feature of an undiagnosed clotting disorder.

86 Postoperative visual loss following non-ocular surgery — Answers: B C D

Postoperative visual loss is thankfully rare, but much less rare following prolonged operations in the prone position. The diagnosis is usually one of ischaemic optic neuropathy. Pressure on the globe can result in blindness, but usually secondary to retinal artery thrombosis. Risk factors are prone position, prolonged surgery, hypotension, large blood loss, and possibly a history of hypertension, diabetes and glaucoma. Although the defect may improve over time it usually doesn't.

Ref: Geeraerts T and Devys J M. Postoperative visual loss following prone spinal surgery. *Br J Anaest* 2005; **95:** 719–720.

87 Electroconvulsive therapy **Answers: B C D E**

ECT can be given without consent, although a second opinion from the Mental Health Commission must state that the treatment is necessary. ECT causes vagal stimulation, and so pre-treatment with glycopyrulate reduces the risk of bradycardia. Methohexitone is an IV induction agent which reduces the seizure threshold, making it ideal for a procedure which aims to provoke seizures. It is no longer available in this country, but is specially imported by some anaesthetists. !!

Without muscle relaxation the provoked seizures can cause fractures, avulsions and dislocations.

88 Transvenous temporary pacemakers for bradycardia **Answers: B C E**

Temporary pacemakers stimulate the right ventricle with a bipolar wire. The pacing output is set 2–3× above the minimal stimulating current. If capture is occurring the pacing box should be kept in VVI (demand) to allow the innate rhythm to take over should recovery occur.

89 Desflurane as compared to isoflurane **Answers: A B**

Isoflurane causes more cardiovascular depression and coronary vasodilation, and they cause about the same amount of muscle relaxation.

If you are totally guessing questions like this where the answer can be 'more', 'less', or 'the same', the odds of being correct will be higher if you chose the option that covers two-thirds of the choices. In this case 'false' enables the correct answer to be 'less' or 'the same'. This thought though should be considered in light of the fact that it can be quite difficult to write plausible 'false' questions, and many MCQs are 'true' heavy.

90 Increased levels of plasma unconjugated bilirubin **Answers: A B C**

High levels of unconjugated bilirubin occur if there is increased production (haemolysis), impaired uptake (Gilbert's syndrome) or impaired conjugation (eg in the newborn). High levels of conjugated bilirubin occur if there is decreased excretion (Dubin-Johnson), hepatocellular disease, intrahepatic cholestasis (biliary cirrhosis, drugs), and extra hepatic cholestasis (stone, strictures, tumours). The jaundice of chronic liver failure is mixed and variable with the possibility of increased unconjugated bilirubin because of reduced uptake, and, classically, increased conjugated bilirubin because of intrahepatic obstruction. **C** could therefore be true or false depending on the view of the person setting the question. The real exam has fewer ambiguous or trick questions than MCQ books tend to contain.

Practice Paper 3: Clinical Viva Answers

Viva 1

Examiner 1

Summarise the case and the possible anaesthetic implications
This is an elderly lady with severe rheumatoid disease and oesophageal reflux.

In view of her reflux she would, if a general anaesthetic was used, require a rapid sequence induction. However, in view of her rheumatoid disease affecting the cervical spine, intubation might be hazardous. A regional technique might therefore be the most appropriate anaesthetic.

Describe the findings on the cervical spine X-ray. What is the significance?
The X-ray reveals subluxation of the atlanto-axial joint. Normally there is no gap between the odontoid peg and the arch of the atlas. Subluxation is present when the distance between the atlas odontoid process in the lateral flexion view is >4 mm in patients over 44 years of age or >3 mm in younger patients.

The problem is that the odontoid peg, which is normally held in position by the strong transverse ligament of the atlas, encroaches on the spinal canal in flexion with the risk of spinal cord compression.

Therefore laryngoscopy must be undertaken with care in rheumatoid patients with evidence of cervical spine disease and atlanto-axial subluxation.

Other problems with the airway in rheumatoid arthritis include:

1. Temporomandibular joint dysfunction which may cause reduced mouth opening rendering intubation difficult.
2. Crico-arytenoid joint arthritis which may produce laryngeal obstruction.

Ref: Fombou F, Thompson J. Anaesthesia for the adult patient with rheumatoid arthritis. *Continuing Education in Anaesthesia, Critical Care and Pain* 2006; **6**(6): 235–239

How would you anaesthetise this lady?
I would opt for a regional technique. The options are:

1. epidural
2. spinal
3. combined spinal and epidural
4. combined sciatic and femoral nerve blocks
5. intravenous regional anaesthesia of the lower limb.

The first three options are probably the most straightforward choices.

Examiner 2

What do you think the diagnosis is?
The findings of widely dilated pupils, tachycardia and convulsions in an unconscious patient who has taken some tablets strongly suggest an overdose of tricyclic anti-depressants.

The blood gases are typical. There is a marked metabolic acidosis (bicarbonate 11.4) and hypokalaemia.

The ECG shows right bundle branch block and left posterior fascicular block (ie bifascicular block). Tricyclics have anticholinergic effects which cause cardiac rhythm disturbances.

What is your management?

ABC
The airway is best secured by endotracheal intubation and artificial ventilation. She is likely to be hypovolaemic and will require intravenous fluids. A large-bore nasogastric tube should be passed after intubation and, after confirmation of its position, activated charcoal should be given. Arrhythmias are a major complication of tricyclic overdose but they often respond to correction of hypoxia, electrolytes (including magnesium) and acidosis (with intravenous bicarbonate is necessary).

Short Cases

Examiner 1

What does the chest X-ray show?
What is the likely underlying diagnosis?
The PA chest X-ray shows a well circumscribed partly calcified mass at the upper left heart border. The lateral chest X-ray shows it to be an anterior mediastinal mass and in view of her history of medication for weakness this suggests that the mass is a thymoma and that the patient has myasthenia gravis.

What is myasthenia gravis?
What medications and other treatments are there for this condition?
Myasthenia gravis is an autoimmune disease in which there are antibodies to the post-synaptic acetylcholine receptor of the neuromuscular junction. It results in weakness mainly of proximal limb, facial and eye muscles. It is associated with other autoimmune conditions and patients may have a thymoma.

Management includes pharmacological treatment. Anticholinesterase drugs such as pyridostigmine increase the level of acetylcholine at the neuromuscular junction. An alternative approach is to use immunosuppressive agents such as azathioprine or steroids. Non-pharmacological treatments include plasmapheresis and thymectomy.

What are the anaesthetic implications of myasthenia gravis?
The main consideration is the response of these patients to muscle relaxants.

They require a much smaller dose of non-depolarising muscle relaxant. By contrast they are resistant to suxamethonium and exhibit unusual and sometimes prolonged blocks.

Examiner 2
Here is a CT scan of the brain of a young man who presented to A&E having been knocked unconscious playing rugby. He was initially lucid after regaining consciousness but then lapsed into coma.

What does the scan show?

The unenhanced CT scan of the brain shows a high density collection in the anterior cranial fossa. These is marked compression and distortion of the left frontal lobe and there is some midline shift to the right side. This high density material is fresh blood. The inner margin is convex and it is limited by the attachment of the dura mater to the frontal bone and the coronal suture. This image is consistent with a diagnosis of extradural haematoma – and this is a neurosurgical emergency.

Describe your initial management of this man in A&E
According to the ATLS guidelines my priorities are:
A airway (with cervical spine control)
B breathing
C circulation (with haemorrhage control)
D dysfunction (neurological assessment, including GCS)
E exposure (to identify all injuries).

The aim is to prevent secondary brain damage by preventing hypoxia and hypotension and then once stabilised to refer the patient to the neurological team for evacuation of the haematoma.

Indications for immediate endotracheal intubation and ventilation after head injury are:

1. GCS ≤8
2. Ventilatory insufficiency
   (a) P_aO_2 <9 kPa on air or <13 kPa with O_2
   (b) P_aCO_2 >6 kPa
3. Loss of protective laryngeal reflexes
4. Respiratory arrhythmia
5. Spontaneous hyperventilation causing P_aCO_2 <3.5 kPa

Intubation must be carried out with cervical spine control in case of a coexisting cervical spine injury. A rapid sequence induction should be performed. Thiopentone is the induction agent of choice as it is also an anticonvulsant and reduces cerebral metabolism. A short-acting opioid will reduce the pressor response to laryngoscopy and intubation.

Two large bore (14-G) IV cannulae should be inserted and appropriate fluids given as necessary.

Cerebral perfusion pressure (CPP) equals mean arterial pressure (MAP) minus intracranial pressure (ICP); in this patient a MAP of 90 mmHg should be maintained. Ideally ICP monitoring should be instigated.

There should be a full neurological assessment including the GCS and full exposure of the patient to check for other injuries.

An arterial line to monitor blood pressure and blood gases would be useful.

The P_aO_2 should be kept above 13 kPa and the P_aCO_2 4–4.5 kPa.

Pulse oximetry, ECG, end-tidal CO_2 and urine output should be monitored, as well as regular neurological observations and fluid balance. The patient must be kept sedated and pain free.

Ref: Gentleman D, Dearden M, Midgley S and Maclean D. Guidelines for resuscitation and transfer of patients with serious head injury. *Br Med J* 1993; **307**(6903):547–552.

Ref: *Recommendations for the transfer of patients with acute head injuries to neurosurgical units*. Neuroanaesthetic Society of Great Britain and Ireland

and the Association of Anaesthetists of Great Britain and Ireland. Dec 1996.

Describe your anaesthetic management of a five-year-old who is bleeding following tonsillectomy 6 h previously

Problems which must be addressed

- Haemorrhage – often the amount is underestimated with possible hypovolaemia.
- Swallowed blood and a full stomach predispose to aspiration.
- Potentially difficult airway with blood obscuring the view at laryngoscopy.
- Residual anaesthetic.
- Frightened child and anxious parents.

Preoperative assessment

- Intravenous access and fluid replacement to ensure normovolaemia with cross-matched blood available.
- Establish whether any anaesthetic difficulties were encountered at the original operation, noting particularly endotracheal tube size.
- Consider emptying the stomach with a nasogastric tube, though this may cause more distress and bleeding; or premedication with atropine and an anti-emetic.

Anaesthetic management

- Ensure adequate resuscitation prior to induction.
- Full monitoring prior to induction on tilting table head down, with effective suction.
- Rapid sequence induction with cricoid pressure, thiopentone and suxamethonium.
- Endotracheal intubation which may require a smaller sized tube than before.
- Maintenance with nitrous oxide, oxygen and isoflurane spontaneously breathing through a T-piece.
- Prior to extubation wash the stomach out via a nasogastric tube.
- Extubate head down on side fully awake.

Postoperatively

- Check Hb.
- Beware of airway obstruction if the throat has been packed or if pre-existing sleep apnoea.
- Consider high dependency unit for close monitoring.

Paper 3 Clinical Sciences Viva Answers

1 Compare and contrast etomidate and ketamine?

In what situations would you use these drugs?

	Etomidate	Ketamine
Chemical	Carboxylated imidazole derivative	Phencyclidine derivative
Presentation	2mg/ml in water with 35% propylene glycol, pH 8.1	10/50/100 mg/ml of a racemic mixture. 50/100 mg/kg have Benzethonium Cl as a preservative
Main action	Hypnotic	Dissociative anaesthesia (analgesia + superficial sleep)
Mode of action	Unknown, only the D-isomer works	Non-competative anatagonist of NMDA receptor Ca channel pore + inhibits NMDA activity by interaction with phencyclidine binding site. May also modulate opiod and muscarinic recepts
Dose	IV 0.3mg/kg, acts in 10-65s, duration 6-8mins	IM 10mg/kg, action in 2-10 mins, dur 10-20mins IV 1.5-2mg/kg, actin in 30s, dur 5-10mins IVI 50mcg/kg/min Extradural – (adult dose 10mg) Intrathecal or oral
Effects	CVS – relatively stable RS - v RR, TV, coughing, hiccups CNS – may cause involuntary musc movements, v ICP, v IOP, vCBF, v metabolic rate AS – nausea in 2-15% (40% if opiate also used) Other – inhibits steroidogenesis, v cortisol and aldosterone for 24hrs after admin	CVS- ^HR, ^BP, ^CVP, ^Cardiac O/P, baroreceptor function maintained, dysrhythmias uncommon RS- mild stimulation, relative preservation reflexes, bronchodilatation CNS- ^ CBF + metabolic rate, ^ IOP, amnesia, EEG dominant theta and loss of alpha rhythm AS- ^salivation, PONV common Other- ^circulation levels catecholamines, ^tone and activity of striated muscle

	Etomidate	Ketamine
Toxicity/ Side-effects	Pain on injection in 25-50%, myoclonus, ^ mortality if used for ITU sedation	transient rash in 15%, emergence delirium/ hallucinations, pain on injection
Kinetics Distribution	76% protein bound, rapid redistribution of bolus	20% oral bioavailability 20-50% protein bound, half life 11mins, recovery mainly due to redistribution
Metabolism	Rapid by plasma and hepatic esterases to inactive metabolites	N-demethlyation and hydroxylation of the cyclohexylamine ring in the liver, some active products
Excretion	87% in urine (3% unchanges)	conjugated metabolites in urine
Special points	Porphyrinogenic in animal models A lipid formulation is less irritant on injection	emergence problems less in young and old, with quiet recovery, with opiates and benzos antisialogogue recommended
Uses	IV induction in situations where CVS stability is particularly important	i) IV induction, esp in high risk patients ii) sole agent for short procedures iii) anaesthesia in the field iv) periop analgesia v) chronic pain management vi) induction critically ill children and asthma

2 What is a laser?

What types of laser do you know and what are they used for?

What safety precautions are necessary?

Laser = Light Amplification of Stimulated Emission of Radiation

Laser light is

Monochromatic - has a narrow wavelength band

Coherent: Oscillate in phase so all peaks and troughs are in the same position

Collimated : Do not disperse

Components

Medium (compound to release photons, can be gas or solid)

Mirror (one of which is only partially reflective to allow escape of 1% of the light)

Pump (energy source)

Types of Laser

- CO_2 is long infra red light 10600nm and is absorbed rapidly by water giving explosive vaporisation of cells close to the surface. Used for cutting and debulking
- Nd-YAG is short infrared 1064nm and is absorbed slower by water so penetrates deeper and heats slower causing coagulation.
- Ruby 694nm is absorbed by dark pigmented tissue
- Argon 500,000nm is absorbed by red tissue (vascular). Used to coagulate small vessels e.g. ophthalmology

Safety

- Protective eyewear from direct and reflected light
- Non reflective instruments
- Danger of fire: avoid alcohol, non flammable ET tube and volatile agent
- Danger of damage to tube cuff, use double cuff and fill with saline

3 Describe the anatomy of the lumbar plexus.

Describe how you would perform a lumbar plexus block.

Lumbar plexus is formed by the ventral rami of the first three lumbar nerves (occasionally with a contribution from T12) and the greater part of the 4th that unite to form the following nerves: iliohypogastric (L1), ilio-inguinal (L1), genitofemoral (L1/2), lateral femoral cutaneous (L2/3), femoral nerve (L2,3,4), and obturator (L2,3,4). The plexus is located in a virtual space in the psoas major muscle.

The block is performed with the patient in the lateral position with hips and knees flexed to 90°, the side to be blocked uppermost. In an adult the needle insertion point is approximately 4cm lateral to the spinal process of L4.

A landmark method is used. The line joining the top of the iliac crests normally crosses a line made by joining the superior iliac crests at L4/L5 level. Having identified L4, a line parallel to the spinous processes is drawn which passes through the post superior iliac spine. The insertion point is 2/3 of the distance from the spinous process of L4 along a perpendicular line joining L4 and the line passing through the post superior iliac spine.

An insulated nerve stimulator needle is introduced perpendicularly to skin through muscle until it reaches the transverse process of L4 . The insertion depth is noted and the needle withdrawn slightly and reorientated with a 5° angle in cephalic or caudal direction (to avoid transverse process). The needle is inserted more deeply (to a maximum of 20mm more) until the required stimulation of the femoral nerve (ascension of the patella) can be observed. After check aspiration a single injection of e.g. 30mls of 0.375% bupivicaine is given.

4 Describe the effects mediated by the different types of adrenergic receptors. Give examples of drugs that act at these receptors.

Adrenergic receptors

- Alpha receptors
  - Post-synaptic cardiac alpha$_1$ receptors – stimulation causes increase in contractility without increase in heart rate; not mediated by camp; effect more pronounced at low heart rates; slower onset and longer duration than beta$_1$ receptor mediated response
  - Pre-synaptic alpha$_2$ receptors in heart and vasculature – activated by norepinephrine released by sympathetic nerve itself and mediates negative feedback inhibition of further norepinephrine release
  - Post-synaptic alpha1 and alpha$_2$ receptors in peripheral vessels mediate vasoconstriction
- Beta receptors
  - Post-synaptic beta$_1$ receptors – predominant adrenergic receptors in the heart; stimulation causes increased rate and force of contraction; mediated by cAMP
  - Post-synaptic beta$_2$ receptors – in vasculature mediate vasodilatation; smooth muscle relaxation

Adrenergic agonists

- Adrenaline – stimulates alpha$_1$<beta$_2$<beta$_1$; effects mediated by stimulation of adenyl cyclase leading to increase in cAMP

    - Used to increase haemodynamic and oxygen transport variables e.g. in septic patients to supranormal levels
- Noradrenaline – alpha and beta$_1$ agonist with no clinically significant beta$_2$ effects
    - Equipotent with adrenaline as a beta$_1$ agonist but less potent an alpha agonist in most tissues
    - Used for refractory hypotension
- Ephedrine – naturally occurring amine with both direct and indirect sympathomimetic effects; stimulates noradrenaline release from post ganglionic sympathetic nerve endings
- Isoproterenol (isoprenaline) – powerful non-selective beta agonist with virtually no alpha effects
- Salbutamol - beta$_2$ agonist
- Metaraminol – alpha and beta agonist with direct and indirect effects (similar to ephedrine but overall peripheral resistance is increased, thus greater increase in BP, especially diastolic BP)
- Methoxamine – direct and indirect effects; alpha agonist and beta blocker; primary effect is peripheral vasoconstriction
- Phenylephrine – direct acting, potent alpha and weak beta agonist, similar effects to noradrenaline
- Phosphodiesterase inhibitors (eg. Enoximone) – inhibits phophodiesterase in cardiac tissue thus increasing intracellular cAMP (phosphodiesterase inactivates it) and increasing intracellular calcium availability by causing increased calcium influx via slow channel; this increases rate and force of myocardial contraction
    - cAMP also affects diastolic heart function through the regulation of phospholamban (regulatory subunit of Ca pump of the sarcoplasmic reticulum – enhances Ca re-sequestration and hence improves diastolic relaxation)
    - Also relaxes vascular smooth muscle – vasodilatation
    - Myocardial oxygen consumption not increased

Short Answer Question Paper 4

1. What bedside tests are available to predict difficult intubation? (70%) Comment on the usefulness of each test. (30%)

2. You are asked to assess a 30-year-old woman complaining of a headache 24 h after having had a lumbar epidural catheter inserted for the provision of analgesia during labour.

   What are the principal differential diagnoses? (20%) What factors would make post dural puncture headache (PDPH) most likely? (30%) How can the patient with PDPH be managed? (50%)

3. A 19-year-old with acute severe asthma presents to your casualty department. How would you make a clinical assessment of the severity of the attack? (50%) What are the indications for mechanical ventilation? (25%) What strategies would you employ to ventilate this patient and why? (25%)

4. What is latex allergy? (30%) Who is at risk of developing latex allergy? (20%) How would you manage a 55-year-old with latex allergy for a check cystoscopy? (50%)

5. A 5-year-old boy is brought into the emergency room after being rescued from a pond. The monitor shows fine ventricular fibrillation. Describe your resuscitation including relevant drugs, with doses, and equipment sizes.

6. Discuss the principles of management of a 35-year-old patient with myasthenia gravis who requires a thymectomy.

7. What are the specific problems associated with anaesthesia for elective surgery in the patient with dialysis-dependent renal failure?

8. Describe the principles involved in the pulse oximetry. (50%) What are its limitations in clinical practice? (50%)

9. Describe the nerve supply to the foot. (40%) How would you perform an ankle block? (60%)

10. Summarise the peri-operative management of a 55-year-old with a body mass index of 38 kg·m^{-2} who requires a laparoscopic cholecystectomy.

11. How may homologous blood transfusion be minimised peri-operatively?

12. What are the options for pain relief following a thoracotomy? (40%) What are the advantages and disadvantages of each? (60%)

Multiple Choice Question Paper 4

1 Magnetic resonance imaging

❑ A the magnetic field causes alignment of tissue atom nuclei with even numbers of protons or neutrons
❑ B radiofrequency pulses cause deflection of the aligned atom nuclei, and absorption of energy that is released when the atom nuclei return to alignment
❑ C flowing blood shows up brightly (white) on T_1-weighted scans
❑ D is better than CT at visualising the posterior fossa of the skull
❑ E only coronal images can be viewed

2 Infrared spectrophotometry can be used to measure the following

❑ A oxygen
❑ B carbon dioxide
❑ C helium
❑ D isoflurane
❑ E nitrous oxide

3 The Clarke oxygen electrode

❑ A requires a power source
❑ B the anode is made of lead
❑ C the key reaction is reduction of oxygen at the cathode
❑ D may be inaccurate in the presence of nitrous oxide
❑ E is maintained at 37°C

4 The reading of the pulse oximeter can be unreliable in the following circumstances

❑ A carboxyhaemoglobin
❑ B fetal haemoglobin
❑ C sickle cell disease
❑ D polycythaemia
❑ E anaemia

5 The Tec6 desflurane vaporiser

- ❑ A is heated to overcome the low saturated vapour pressure
- ❑ B is colour-coded purple
- ❑ C has an alarm to warn against running low on volatile
- ❑ D with necessary connectors could be used within the breathing circuit
- ❑ E contains a pressure transducer

6 Cardiorespiratory exercise (CPX) testing

- ❑ A evaluates cardiac and respiratory function
- ❑ B subjects exercise against a fixed level of resistance
- ❑ C exercise-induced cardiac ischaemia can also be diagnosed
- ❑ D the anaerobic threshold (AT) is determined from a plot of VCO_2 vs VO_2
- ❑ E patients with an AT of <11 ml/min per kg have a high risk of perioperative mortality

7 Concerning fetal monitoring during labour

- ❑ A a baseline heart rate 110–150 beats/min with a variability of 5–25 is normal
- ❑ B a loss of baseline variability may reflect fetal hypoxia
- ❑ C a loss of baseline variability may reflect fetal sleep
- ❑ D early decelerations reflect fetal hypoxia
- ❑ E a fetal scalp blood pH of 7.3 warrants immediate delivery

8 The oesophageal Doppler

- ❑ A can give a continuous measure of cardiac output
- ❑ B measures the velocity of blood in the ascending aorta
- ❑ C relies upon the phase shift from transmitted to reflected ultrasound
- ❑ D an FTc of 350–400 is optimal
- ❑ E the probe can be inserted nasally

9 The bispectral index (BIS) monitor

- ❑ A the probability of recall is very low if the BIS is kept <60
- ❑ B BIS demonstrates a dose–response effect with isoflurane
- ❑ C BIS demonstrates a dose–response effect with midazolam
- ❑ D BIS demonstrates a dose–response effect with ketamine
- ❑ E use generally results in more anaesthetic agents being used

10 Intracranial pressure monitoring

- ❑ A the normal pressure in supine adults is 7–15 mmHg (1–2 kPa)
- ❑ B the pressure trace resembles the arterial waveform
- ❑ C extradural fibre optic probes have the lowest infection rates
- ❑ D the pressure falls with each ventilator-delivered breath
- ❑ E A waves are a reassuring sign

11 A fixed cardiac output state can occur with

- ❑ A constrictive pericarditis
- ❑ B mitral stenosis
- ❑ C patent ductus arteriosus
- ❑ D aortic stenosis
- ❑ E hypertrophic obstructive cardiomyopathy

12 Ulcerative colitis

- ❑ A is associated with cirrhosis
- ❑ B is associated with finger clubbing
- ❑ C is associated with cholangitis
- ❑ D is associated with carcinoma of the colon
- ❑ E rarely responds to steroids

13 Obstructive jaundice

- ❑ A causes high circulating levels of unconjugated bilirubin
- ❑ B leads to a high faecal fat level
- ❑ C is associated with an alkaline phosphatase level >100 IU/l
- ❑ D leads to a high level of urobilinogen in the blood
- ❑ E may cause a coagulopathy

14 A raised reticulocyte count is found in

- ❑ A untreated megaloblastic anaemia
- ❑ B untreated iron deficiency
- ❑ C congenital spherocytosis
- ❑ D sickle cell trait
- ❑ E haemolysis

15 Mitral stenosis is associated with

- ❑ A a loud first heart sound
- ❑ B an early diastolic murmur
- ❑ C a displaced apex beat
- ❑ D a malar flush
- ❑ E atrial fibrillation

16 Vomiting may be associated with

- ❑ A metabolic alkalosis
- ❑ B alkaline urine
- ❑ C raised plasma chloride levels
- ❑ D hyperkalaemia
- ❑ E elevated blood urea

17 The complications of Crohn's disease include

- ❑ A entero-enteric fistula formation
- ❑ B recurrence following excision of the primary lesion
- ❑ C fistula in ano
- ❑ D lymphoma
- ❑ E polyarthritis

18 Recognised causes of glycosuria include

- ❑ A phaeochromocytoma
- ❑ B pregnancy
- ❑ C partial gastrectomy
- ❑ D hypopituitarism
- ❑ E subarachnoid haemorrhage

19 Complications of long-term spironolactone therapy include

- ❑ A metabolic alkalosis
- ❑ B hyponatraemia
- ❑ C hypoglycaemia
- ❑ D hyperkalaemia
- ❑ E hyperuricaemia

20 In patients with untreated megaloblastic anaemia

- ❑ A histamine fast achlorhydria is always present
- ❑ B there may be a peripheral neuropathy
- ❑ C there is an increased incidence of carcinoma of the stomach
- ❑ D resection of the ileum for Crohn's disease may be causally related
- ❑ E the serum B12 level may be within the normal range

21 Estimation of prothrombin time is useful in

- ❑ A haemophilia
- ❑ B von Willebrand's disease
- ❑ C scurvy
- ❑ D jaundice
- ❑ E thrombocytopenic purpura

22 Cataract may be caused by

- ❑ A ageing
- ❑ B diabetes mellitus
- ❑ C dystrophia myotonica
- ❑ D electric shock
- ❑ E thyrotoxicosis

23 The generic pacemaker code

- ❑ A position 1 signifies the chamber paced
- ❑ B a 'D' in position 2 means both chambers are sensed
- ❑ C an 'I' in position 3 means the pacemaker will trigger in response to a ventricular contraction
- ❑ D position 4 signifies the response to a bradycardia
- ❑ E position 5 defines the available functions for tachycardias (eg none, pacing, shock)

24 Pneumothorax

- ❑ A may be caused by a severe cough
- ❑ B is associated with emphysema
- ❑ C may appear post thyroidectomy
- ❑ D is best diagnosed with a supine, inspiratory chest X-ray
- ❑ E 70% N_2O can double the size of the pneumothorax in 10 min

25 Oesophageal atresia

- ❑ A about 20% will also have tracheo-oesophageal fistula
- ❑ B face mask ventilation is contraindicated
- ❑ C may present with recurrent pneumonia
- ❑ D diagnosis is by contrast radiology
- ❑ E surgical correction of fistulae is usually possible via a cervical incision

26 The thalassaemias

- ❑ A adults with α thalassaemia have increased amounts of fetal haemoglobin (HbF)
- ❑ B α/α+ is 'silent'
- ❑ C β thalassaemia minor (β/β+) is characterised by anaemia (Hb <9 g/dl) and splenomegaly
- ❑ D the aim of transfusion therapy is to keep Hb >9 g/dl
- ❑ E desferrioxamine should be avoided as iron overload causes cardiac toxicity

27 Autonomic neuropathy

- ❑ A can cause delayed gastric emptying
- ❑ B can cause cardiac conduction defects
- ❑ C occurs in diabetes mellitus
- ❑ D occurs in Guillain-Barré syndrome
- ❑ E is indicated by a postural systolic BP drop of 30 mmHg

28 Developmental milestones

- ❑ A a 3-month-old baby is able to smile
- ❑ B a child of 12 months should understand 'get your shoes'
- ❑ C most children walk by the age of 18 months
- ❑ D it is normal for a mother not to understand her 2½-year-old child's speech most of the time
- ❑ E a child of 3½ uses a vocabulary of about 50 words

29 Amphotericin B

- ❑ A is an antifungal antibiotic
- ❑ B is used to treat allergic bronchopulmonary aspergillosis
- ❑ C is nephrotoxic
- ❑ D is given as a bolus dose
- ❑ E may cause arrhythmias

30 Acute cholecystitis

- ❑ A follows impaction of a gallstone in the cystic duct
- ❑ B classically Murphy's sign is positive
- ❑ C does not cause jaundice
- ❑ D abdominal ultrasound can aid in diagnosis
- ❑ E may be treated by early cholecystectomy

31 The specific gravity of urine is reduced in

- ❑ A diabetes insipidus
- ❑ B acute tubular necrosis
- ❑ C intestinal obstruction
- ❑ D lithium toxicity
- ❑ E diabetes mellitus

32 Cardiac tamponade

- ❑ A may complicate aortic dissection
- ❑ B produces a rise in jugular venous pressure
- ❑ C causes a small radial pulse which fades on inspiration
- ❑ D is different from congestive cardiac failure (CCF) in not causing hepatomegaly
- ❑ E is best treated by a vigorous diuretic regime

33 Propranolol administered intravenously

- ❑ A decreases airway resistance
- ❑ B causes hyperglycaemia
- ❑ C decreases the inotropic action of digitalis
- ❑ D is dangerous in patients receiving verapamil
- ❑ E is the agent of choice for the treatment of ventricular ectopic beats in a patient with an acute myocardial infarct

34 Concerning the 2005 Resuscitation Council guidelines on adult defibrillation

- ❑ A when using a monophasic defibrillator the first shock should be at 200 J
- ❑ B when using a monophasic defibrillator all subsequent shocks should be at 360 J
- ❑ C the minimum energy level when using a biphasic defibrillator is 200 J
- ❑ D biphasic defibrillators are able to compensate for variations in thoracic bioimpedance
- ❑ E the biphasic truncated exponential waveform is more efficacious than the rectilinear biphasic waveform

35 Following massive blood transfusion

- ❑ A citrate toxicity causes a metabolic acidosis
- ❑ B low levels of 2,3-DPG cause a right shift of the oxyhaemoglobin dissociation curve
- ❑ C metabolic acidosis occurs due to a release of lactic acid from red blood cells
- ❑ D hypothermia causes a right shift in the oxyhaemoglobin dissociation curve
- ❑ E the commonest cause of acidosis is citric acid anticoagulant in the donor blood

36 Intrinsic PEEP

- ❑ A occurs in COPD patients due to dynamic hyperinflation
- ❑ B causes asynchrony of inspiratory muscle activity and inspiratory airflow in the spontaneously breathing patient.
- ❑ C causes the inspiratory muscles to work at a mechanically advantageous shorter length
- ❑ D increases both the resistive and elastic work of breathing
- ❑ E can be reduced by the application of external PEEP during patient-triggered mechanical ventilation

37 Aspiration of gastric contents

- ❑ A is more common following non-anaesthetic emergency intubations than following anaesthesia for emergency surgery
- ❑ B is implicated in the pathogenesis of nosocomial pneumonia
- ❑ C is increased when patients on ITU are nursed semi-recumbent rather than supine
- ❑ D high-volume low-pressure endotracheal tube cuffs allow a greater degree of aspiration than low-volume high-pressure cuffs
- ❑ E Large-bore nasogastric tubes increase the risk of aspiration in ITU patients

38 The following initial ventilator settings are suitable for ventilating a patient with acute severe bronchospasm

- ❑ A V_T ~ 10–15 ml/kg
- ❑ B Respiratory rate 15–20 breaths/min
- ❑ C Inverse ratio ventilation I:E ratio 2:1
- ❑ D Peak inspiratory flow rate >100 l/min
- ❑ E PEEP 10 cmH_2O

39 Concerning scoring systems in ITU

- ❑ A the updated APACHE II scoring system uses more physiological variables than the previous APACHE I scoring system
- ❑ B the APACHE II score uses the worst values of physiological variables in the first hour of ICU stay
- ❑ C the higher the APACHE II score the higher the risk of hospital death
- ❑ D the Simplified Acute Physiology System (SAPS), unlike APACHE II, does not include any scoring for underlying chronic clinical conditions
- ❑ E the Therapeutic Intervention Scoring System (TISS) is scored within the first 24 h of ICU stay

40 The troponins

- ❑ A can be detected in serum 7 days after myocardial infarction
- ❑ B are more sensitive than CK-MB in diagnosis of myocardial infarction
- ❑ C are significantly elevated in serum within 1 h of myocardial infarction
- ❑ D when detected in serum invariably reflect irreparable myocardial damage
- ❑ E have a prognostic role in critical illness

41 Hyperbaric oxygen therapy

- ❑ A causes vasodilatation in normal tissues
- ❑ B reduces the effects of catecholamines
- ❑ C stimulates angiogenesis in radiation-damaged tissues
- ❑ D causes a fall in mixed venous oxygen saturations
- ❑ E may result in hyperglycaemia

42 The following are factors increasing the risk of nosocomial infection

- ❑ A malnutrition
- ❑ B renal failure
- ❑ C poor hand hygiene
- ❑ D gastric pH <4
- ❑ E antibiotic therapy

43 The following antibiotics are bacteriostatic

- ❑ A penicillin
- ❑ B cefuroxime
- ❑ C erythromycin
- ❑ D metronidazole
- ❑ E fluconazole

44 Basal daily requirements for a healthy 80-kg man are approximately

- ❑ A calcium 100 mmol
- ❑ B sodium 100 mmol
- ❑ C potassium 100 mmol
- ❑ D magnesium 100 mmol
- ❑ E phosphate 100 mmol

45 Enteral nutrition for the ITU patient

- ❑ A reduces the risk of stress ulcers
- ❑ B reduces bacterial translocation
- ❑ C increases the incidence of acute cholecystitis
- ❑ D is associated with a low incidence of diarrhoea
- ❑ E should be stopped if bowel sounds are absent

46 Triage priority at a major incident

- ❑ A walking wounded are labelled for urgent treatment
- ❑ B a patient with a clear airway who is not breathing needs immediate treatment
- ❑ C capillary refill of >2 s needs immediate treatment
- ❑ D disability can be assessed on the AVPU scale
- ❑ E only a doctor may pronounce death on scene

47 Treatment of cyanide poisoning may include

- ❑ A sodium nitrite
- ❑ B sodium thiosulphate
- ❑ C sodium nitroprusside
- ❑ D dicobalt edetate
- ❑ E hydroxocobalamin

48 Indications for early intubation of burn patients

- ❑ A stridor
- ❑ B facial burns caused by steam
- ❑ C circumferential burns of the neck
- ❑ D 45% carboxyhaemoglobinaemia
- ❑ E full thickness burns of the nose

49 Clinical features of fulminant hepatic failure include

- ❑ A encephalopathy
- ❑ B impaired platelet function
- ❑ C hyperdynamic circulation
- ❑ D hypoglycaemia
- ❑ E sepsis

50 Complications associated with total parenteral nutrition (TPN) include

- ❑ A hyperglycaemia
- ❑ B hypophosphataemia
- ❑ C metabolic acidosis
- ❑ D hypernatraemia
- ❑ E trace element deficiency

51 Regarding severe pre-eclampsia

- ❑ A magnesium sulphate is the anticonvulsant of choice
- ❑ B there may be a coagulopathy
- ❑ C normal vaginal delivery is usually possible
- ❑ D intravenous fluids are rarely necessary
- ❑ E general anaesthesia is the preferred type of anaesthetic if a caesarean section is required

52 Suxamethonium is contraindicated

- ❑ A in acute renal failure
- ❑ B in Creutzfeldt–Jakob disease
- ❑ C in dystrophia myotonica
- ❑ D in acute intermittent porphyria
- ❑ E the day after spinal cord injury

53 A thyroid storm may require treatment with

- ❑ A diazepam
- ❑ B propranolol
- ❑ C paracetamol
- ❑ D verapamil
- ❑ E chlorpromazine

54 The following anaesthetic agents are safe in a patient with acute porphyria

- ❑ A methohexitone
- ❑ B suxamethonium
- ❑ C diazepam
- ❑ D propofol
- ❑ E isoflurane

55 Sensory signs may occur with

- ❑ A carpal tunnel syndrome
- ❑ B tabes dorsalis
- ❑ C syringomyelia
- ❑ D motor neurone disease
- ❑ E multiple sclerosis

56 Phantom limb pain

- ❑ A can be worsened by spinal anaesthesia
- ❑ B is worse if the limb is painful prior to amputation
- ❑ C incidence is reduced if an amputation is performed under neuraxial block
- ❑ D is effectively treated by systemic opioids
- ❑ E rarely responds to any form of therapy

57 A retrobulbar block will block the following

- ❑ A short ciliary nerves
- ❑ B optic nerves
- ❑ C abducent nerve
- ❑ D facial nerve
- ❑ E oculomotor nerve

58 To suture a laceration on the palm of the hand the following should be blocked

❑ A median nerve
❑ B ulnar nerve
❑ C musculocutaneous nerve
❑ D radial nerve
❑ E axillary nerve

59 Coronary artery blood flow

❑ A occurs mainly in diastole
❑ B is autoregulated
❑ C is reduced by tachycardia
❑ D accounts for about 5% of the cardiac output
❑ E is reduced if the venous pressure falls

60 The following drugs cross the blood–brain barrier

❑ A L-Dopa
❑ B atropine
❑ C neostigmine
❑ D mannitol
❑ E fentanyl

61 The speed of uptake of an anaesthetic agent from the lung

❑ A is proportional to the cardiac output
❑ B is proportional to the minute ventilation
❑ C is proportional to the minimum alveolar concentration
❑ D is proportional to the blood gas solubility
❑ E is temperature dependent

62 Ketamine

❑ A has minimal analgesic properties
❑ B may provoke bronchospasm
❑ C is an antagonist at the NMDA receptor
❑ D is presented as a racemic mixture
❑ E is an appropriate agent for the induction of patients with haemorrhagic shock

63 Complications of supraclavicular brachial plexus block include

- ❑ A Horner's syndrome
- ❑ B phrenic nerve paralysis
- ❑ C recurrent laryngeal nerve paralysis
- ❑ D subclavian artery puncture
- ❑ E subarachnoid injection of local anaesthetic solution

64 In axillary brachial plexus block

- ❑ A the lateral cutaneous nerve of the forearm may be unaffected
- ❑ B the phrenic nerve may be damaged
- ❑ C there is a risk of pneumothorax
- ❑ D Horner's syndrome may occur
- ❑ E the shoulder muscles may be paralysed

65 Concerning intercostal block at the posterior angle of the ribs

- ❑ A the local anaesthetic will spread to segments above and below the site of injection
- ❑ B bilateral blocks should not be performed
- ❑ C the local anaesthetic should be injected between the internal and the innermost intercostal muscles
- ❑ D sympathetic blockade is a recognised complication
- ❑ E addition of adrenaline is contraindicated

66 Concerning caudal anaesthesia

- ❑ A there is no risk of dural puncture
- ❑ B the fetal head may be punctured when performed in labour
- ❑ C the volume of local anaesthetic required to block one segment is the same as that required in the lumbar region
- ❑ D a catheter technique cannot be used
- ❑ E the failure rate is higher than for lumbar epidural block

67 Epidural test doses are used to

- ❑ A speed onset of analgesia
- ❑ B detect subarachnoid injection
- ❑ C prevent neurological complications
- ❑ D prevent tachyphylaxis
- ❑ E detect intravenous injection

68 Concerning pacemakers and anaesthesia

- ❑ A induction of anaesthesia may alter pacemaker function
- ❑ B unipolar diathermy should be used
- ❑ C a patient with a pacemaker may safely enter an MRI scanner
- ❑ D postoperative shivering may affect pacemaker function
- ❑ E a magnet placed over a demand pacemaker will convert it to a fixed-rate pacemaker

69 Concerning Moffet's solution

- ❑ A it contains cocaine at a concentration of 100 mg/ml
- ❑ B it contains adrenaline at a concentration of 0.1 mg/ml
- ❑ C it may lead to ventricular fibrillation in occasional patients
- ❑ D the safe maximum dose for cocaine to the nasal mucosa is 15 mg/kg
- ❑ E it is used to improve postoperative analgesia

70 A post-partum headache may be caused by

- ❑ A post dural puncture headache
- ❑ B subarachnoid haemorrhage
- ❑ C cephalgia fugax
- ❑ D cortical vein thrombosis
- ❑ E herpes simplex encephalitis

71 Concerning a Bier's block

- ❑ A 0.5% bupivacaine is a suitable agent
- ❑ B the tourniquet may be deflated safely after 10 min
- ❑ C the tourniquet should be inflated to 100 mmHg above systolic blood pressure
- ❑ D prilocaine may cause carboxyhaemoglobinaemia
- ❑ E a double tourniquet must be used

72 Possible complications of a caudal epidural block include

- ❑ A motor blockade
- ❑ B delayed micturition
- ❑ C subarachnoid block
- ❑ D infection
- ❑ E cauda equina syndrome

73 Complex regional pain syndrome type 1 (reflex sympathetic dystrophy)

- ❑ A may be treated with guanethidine blocks
- ❑ B is associated with allodynia
- ❑ C is associated with hyperalgesia
- ❑ D is associated with osteoporosis of the affected limb
- ❑ E causes purely sensory dysfunction

74 In the *Report on Confidential Enquiries into Maternal Deaths in the United Kingdom 2000–2002*

- ❑ A maternal mortality is about 1 in 10 000
- ❑ B haemorrhage was the commonest cause of death
- ❑ C the percentage of deaths due to anaesthesia increased from the previous report
- ❑ D all the anaesthetic-related deaths were associated with general anaesthesia
- ❑ E most deaths due to anaesthesia were due to airway problems

75 Intrathecal opioids

- ❑ A may cause urinary retention
- ❑ B may cause shivering
- ❑ C may produce total spinal blockade
- ❑ D may produce pruritus, relieved by propofol
- ❑ E are unlikely to produce significant respiratory depression

76 Concerning nitrous oxide

- ❑ A the cylinder pressure is 137 bar
- ❑ B the filling ratio is 0.67
- ❑ C the cylinder pressure falls linearly with use
- ❑ D the critical temperature is –8°C
- ❑ E it can cause vitamin B_{12} deficiency

77 The minimum alveolar concentration (MAC) of a volatile agent

- ❑ A decreases with increasing age
- ❑ B is increased in pregnancy
- ❑ C is greater in men than in women
- ❑ D is greater in neonates than in infants of 2 years of age
- ❑ E is reduced at altitude

78 In one-lung anaesthesia the partial pressure of oxygen in the blood depends on

- ❑ A the inspired oxygen tension
- ❑ B the intraoperative haematocrit
- ❑ C the mixed venous oxygen tension
- ❑ D the amount of blood flow to the unventilated lung
- ❑ E the cardiac output

79 Concerning the Mapleson classification of breathing systems

- ❑ A the Bain system is a Mapleson D system
- ❑ B the Mapleson A system is the most efficient for spontaneous ventilation
- ❑ C there are no valves in the Mapleson E breathing system
- ❑ D all the systems are partial rebreathing systems
- ❑ E the Bain system may be used with some ventilators

80 In a patient taking 10 mg of prednisolone daily for rheumatoid arthritis

- ❑ A the steroid should be omitted on the day of operation
- ❑ B excessive doses of glucocorticosteroids increase susceptibility to infection
- ❑ C glucocorticosteroids are needed for the response to surgical stress
- ❑ D the circulating plasma cortisol concentration is normal by 1–2 days after surgical stress in most patients
- ❑ E supplementary hydrocortisone should be given in the peri-operative period

81 The following are an indication for oxygen therapy

- ❑ A carbon monoxide poisoning
- ❑ B haemorrhagic shock
- ❑ C acute asthma attack
- ❑ D diffusion hypoxia
- ❑ E retrolental fibroplasia

82 Concerning the Apgar score

- ❑ A it is valid in coloured babies
- ❑ B it is measured 1 min after delivery of the head
- ❑ C it is a sensitive indicator of fetal distress
- ❑ D heart rate is as important as skin colour
- ❑ E muscle tone is not assessed

83 Mannitol

- ❑ A is a sugar
- ❑ B is useful before biliary surgery
- ❑ C may cause circulatory overload
- ❑ D may cause neurological deterioration
- ❑ E is found in commercial preparations of dantrolene

84 Negative nitrogen balance is found in

- ❑ A acute renal failure
- ❑ B post surgery
- ❑ C cortisone therapy
- ❑ D pregnancy
- ❑ E starvation

85 An asthmatic patient becomes wheezy towards the end of an anaesthetic; contributory factors may include

- ❑ A irritation of the trachea by an endotracheal tube
- ❑ B use of neostigmine
- ❑ C use of isoflurane
- ❑ D light anaesthesia
- ❑ E intravenous morphine

86 Pregnancy is associated with

- ❑ A reduced functional residual capacity
- ❑ B reduced vital capacity
- ❑ C increased airway resistance
- ❑ D increased alveolar ventilation
- ❑ E a hypercoagulable state

87 Predisposing factors for pre-eclampsia include

- ❑ A primagravida
- ❑ B teenage pregnancy
- ❑ C twin pregnancy
- ❑ D migraine
- ❑ E chronic hypertension

88 Advantages of regional technique for transurethral resection of prostate

- ❑ A bladder perforation more easily recognised
- ❑ B reduced incidence of DVT
- ❑ C increased patient dignity
- ❑ D patient avoidance of teratogens
- ❑ E reduced incidence of postoperative headache

89 Anaphylactic reactions associated with anaesthesia

- ❑ A bronchospasm is by far the most common presenting feature
- ❑ B if asthmatics have a reaction their bronchospasm may be very difficult to treat
- ❑ C the severity of a reaction is likely to be increased if there is neuraxial anaesthesia
- ❑ D serum mast cell tryptase can distinguish between anaphylactoid and anaphylactic reactions
- ❑ E any patient with a suspected anaphylactic reaction should be referred to an allergist

90 Oral hypoglycaemics

- ❑ A sulfonylureas increase insulin secretion
- ❑ B gliclazide is short acting
- ❑ C biguanides increase insulin sensitivity and hepatic gluconeogenesis
- ❑ D metformin may cause dangerous hypoglycaemia in starved patients
- ❑ E acarbose is an α-glucosidase inhibitor

Practice Paper 4: The Clinical Vivas

Viva 1: The Clinical Viva takes place in the morning.

1. You are given a piece of clinical information and you have 10 min to study it.
2. You will spend 20 min with the first examiner, discussing the clinical care of the patient described and how you would anaesthetise for the case.
3. You will then spend 20 min with a second examiner discussing approximately three unrelated clinical scenarios.

Viva 2: The Clinical Science Viva takes place in the afternoon. Two examiners will question you for approximately 15 min each.

Approximately four topics are covered.

A good way to prepare for the viva is to work with a partner. For this reason we have separated the sample questions in this book from the model answers to allow you to work through the viva session before looking at the answers.

Viva 1

Clinical scenario

A 60-year-old ex-miner has been listed for open resection of a sigmoid carcinoma.

He was medically retired from his work 10 years ago because of problems with his breathing, and has been diagnosed with COPD.

His exercise tolerance, which was always limited, has reduced over the last few weeks, and he can now only manage to walk about 50 m on the flat. He is just able to get up a flight of stairs slowly, but has to stop at the top to catch his breath.

He feels more short of breath when he lies flat, and although he has been sleeping with three pillows he finds himself waking at night breathless.

His current medications are salbutamol and Becotide inhalers and oral prednisolone 2 mg which is a recently reduced dose. He has no allergies.

On examination he is tachypnoeic, with a respiratory rate of 30 breaths/min and S_pO_2 92% breathing air. Fine crackles are heard on auscultation of his chest, particularly at the bases.

His ECG and chest X-ray are shown in Fig. 11a and 11b, respectively.

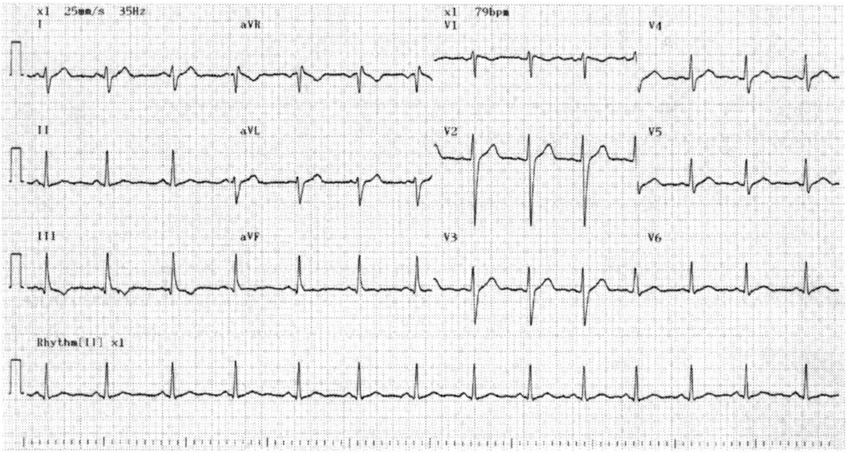

Fig. 11a : Normal ECG

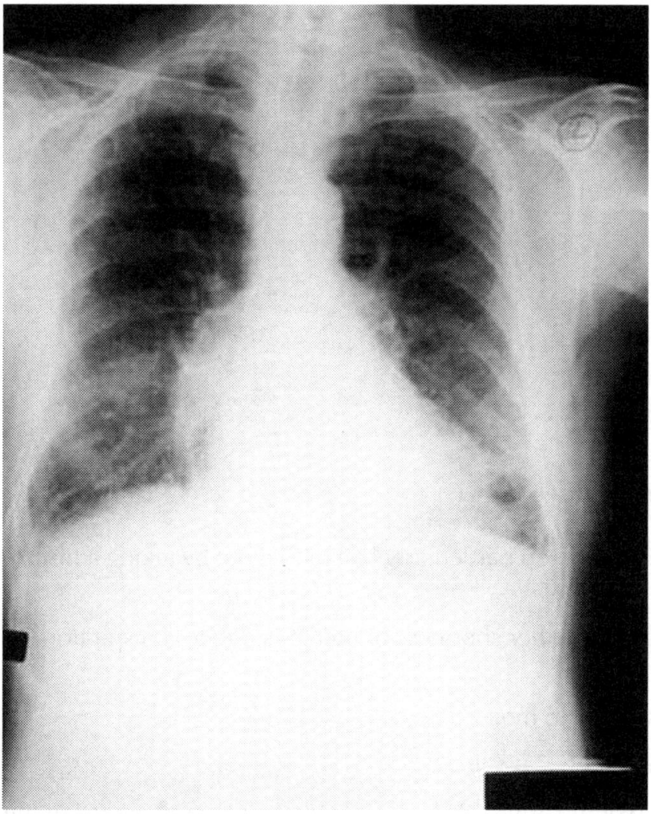

Fig. 10: Chest X-ray (pulmonary fibrosis)

Blood results
Na 141 mmol/l
K 4.2 mmol/l
Urea 5.1 mmol/l
Creatinine 92 μmol/l
Hb 16.0 g/dl
WCC 7.2×10^9/l
plts 402×10^9/l

Arterial blood gas – breathing air

pH	7.39
pCO_2	5.2 kPa
pO_2	10.8 kPa

HCO_3^-	25 mmol	
BE	1.0	

Lung function test

FVC	2.0 litres	50% of predicted
FEV_1	0.7 litres	30%
FEV_1/FVC ratio	43%	
TLC	4.9 litres	93%
VC	2.2 litres	73%
FRC	3.4 litres	104%
RV	2.7 litres	121%
D_LCO	8.6	45%

Examiner 1

Please summarise this case.

What information would you particularly like to find out by taking a history from this patient?

How can you decide whether shortness of breath is due to a respiratory or cardiac cause?

Describe the chest X-ray to me.

Describe the ECG to me.

What do you make of the arterial blood gas? What were you expecting the arterial blood gas to be? How can you explain this arterial blood gas?

Are you ready to anaesthetise him today?

He is now optimised, describe your anaesthetic.

Would you aim to ventilate him postoperatively?

Clinical short cases

Examiner 2

1. You are on-call one Saturday night at your labour ward. There is a commotion in the corridor and a midwife runs up to you and says that an unbooked woman has just been brought in bleeding per vagina.

What is the differential diagnosis?
What do you do first?

The obstetric registrar says she thinks that the woman has placental abruption and needs an emergency caesarean section.

Describe your anaesthetic.
What induction agent would you use for general anaesthesia?
How would you maintain anaesthesia?

2. You have just delivered a fit and well 35-year-old woman to the recovery ward extubated following a straightforward hysterectomy. You are just relaxing in the coffee room when a recovery nurse comes in and says the woman you have just left appears to be very confused.

What would you do?
What is the differential diagnosis?
The recovery staff do an ECG (Fig. 11)
What is your management?

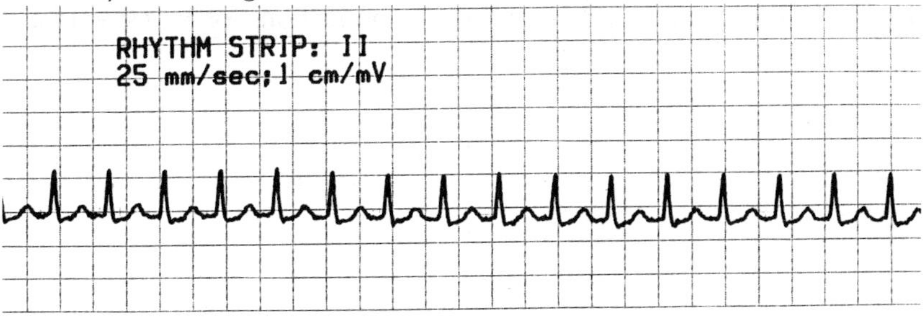

Fig. 11: ECG

3. That afternoon you are anaesthetising for a urology list. The first patient is an 80-year-old man for transurethral resection of a bladder tumour. The surgeon sees you just before you go off to pre-assess the first patient and says that he is worried about the patient moving due to obturator nerve stimulation if you do a regional technique.

What are the anaesthetic options?

Your patient's blood pressure is 180/120 mmHg today.

Would you anaesthetise him today?
How long would you delay the surgery for?

Viva 2

Examiner 1

What is a transducer?
How does an invasive blood pressure transducer work?
Draw a Wheatstone bridge
What are resonance and damping?
What is critical damping and signal-to-noise ratio?

What is the sensory innervation of the head?
What are the branches of the ophthalmic division of the trigeminal nerve?
How might you block them?
What other nerve blocks of the face do you know?

Examiner 2

Tell me about the effects of hypothermia

Please classify antidepressant drugs
For each class explain how they work, their side-effects, what problems they cause in overdose, and if they have special implications for anaesthetists.

SHORT ANSWER QUESTION PAPER 4 ANSWERS

1. What bedside tests are available to predict difficult intubation? (70%) Comment on the usefulness of each test. (30%)

Incidence of difficult intubation is low: ~1:65 of general population with failure to intubate occurring in ~1:2000. Predictive tests therefore need to be both highly sensitive and specific.

There are multiple tests available to predict difficult intubation whose reliability is tested against the ease of intubation classified by Cormack and Lehane, grades I–IV.

(a) Mallampati described a predictive assessment which is made with the patient sitting opposite the assessor. The patient is asked to open the mouth and extend the tongue. The extent to which structures are visible leads to predictive classification.
- Class I: soft palate, faucial pillars and uvula are all visible
- Class II: uvula is obscured by the tongue
- Class III: only the soft palate is visible
- Class IV: added by Sansoon and Young; only the hard palate is seen.

Classes III and IV predict difficult intubation but with low sensitivity of only 50% and specificity of only 4%.

(b) The thyromental distance as described by Patil; if less than 6.5 cm is predictive of difficult intubation, again low sensitivity.

(c) The sternomental distance of less than 12 cm is again predictive of a difficult intubation, with a low sensitivity.

(d) Forward movement of the jaw graded A–C:
- A: lower teeth can protrude further than upper teeth
- B: both sets of teeth meet in the midline
- C: lower teeth cannot reach the upper teeth.

Grades B and C are associated with difficult intubation as the laryngoscope cannot move the jaw anteriorly and the sublingual space is restricted.

(e) Movement of the cervical spine, flexion and extension; most specifically movement at the atlanto-occipital joint. Assessed by placing a finger on the occipital tuberosity and one under the tip of the jaw. The patient is asked to look to the ceiling: normal movement results in the tip of the jaw ending level with or higher than the finger on the occipital tuberosity. Highly sensitive test.

(f) Wilson attempted to improve the sensitivity of the tests by grouping together five factors into a scoring system. The factors are:
- Weight
- Head movements
- Jaw movement
- Mandibular recession
- Buck teeth.

Each factor scores 0, 1 or 2 therefore the maximum score is 10. A score of 2 or more has a sensitivity of 75% of predicting difficult intubation.

Ref: Vaughan R S. Predicting difficult airways. *Br J Anaesth CEPD* 2001; **1** (No 2) April.

Ref: Cobley M and Vaughan R S. Recognition and management of difficult airway problems. *Br J Anaesth* 1992; **68**: 90–97.

2. You are asked to assess a 30-year-old woman complaining of a headache 24 h after having had a lumbar epidural catheter inserted for the provision of analgesia during labour.

What are the principal differential diagnoses? (20%) What factors would make post dural puncture headache (PDPH) most likely? (30%) How can the patient with PDPH be managed? (50%)

Principal differential diagnoses:
- PDPH
- Stress, fatigue and anxiety
- Migraine
- Pre-eclampsia
- Subarachnoid haemorrhage
- Cortical vein thrombosis
- Meningitis, encephalitis
- Sinusitis.

Many PDPH will occur after a recognised dural puncture, though some dural punctures will go unnoticed. The headache of PDP is characteristically positional, worse upright and relieved by recumbency. It is also improved by increasing intra-abdominal and therefore CSF pressure manually. There is no specific distribution within the cranium; the headache may be associated with photophobia, neck stiffness, nausea, diplopia, tinnitus and hearing changes. There is no fever or marked leucocytosis, unlike the infective causes. Focal neurology would indicate some intracranial cause though cranial nerve palsy may occur with PDPH.

Management can be conservative or invasive.

Conservative

1. Hydration. To ensure adequate CSF production, either orally or intravenous infusion.
2. Bed rest. Improves symptoms rather than treatment per se.
3. Non-invasive pressure. Abdominal binders to increase intra-abdominal pressure, which is transmitted to epidural space. Rarely used.
4. Analgesics. Paracetamol, NSAIDs and codeine all help symptoms.
5. Analgesic adjuvants. It is thought that the headache of a PDP is not merely due to low pressure: abnormalities in the cerebral vasculature have also been implicated. Caffeine acts as a cerebral vasoconstrictor and provides good symptomatic relief. Sumatriptan, a 5-HT_1 receptor agonist, has also been used to cause vasoconstriction.

Invasive

1. Epidurally administered fluids if epidural catheter is still in situ, either intermittent boluses or as an infusion. Thought to prevent further CSF leakage and increases the pressure in the epidural space. Variable efficacy.
2. Autologous blood patching is 'Gold standard' treatment: 70–90% PDPH resolve with one patch, 95% with a second patch. Two-operator technique ensures sterility of both the autologous blood and the operator locating the epidural space. Complications include those associated with relocating the epidural space, including dural puncture, meningeal irritation, cranial nerve palsy, raised core body temperature and seizures. These are rare. Prior to blood patching a screen for markers of infection is performed: white cell count and temperature should both be normal and blood should also be sent for microbiological growth.
   As part of the procedure, 5–30 ml of blood is injected, the volume limited by pain presumably due to pressure on the nerve roots. Following the procedure patient should lie still for 2 h.

Ref: Sharpe P. Accidental dural puncture in obstetrics. *Br J Anaesth CEPD Review* 2001; **1**: 81–84.

3. A 19-year-old with acute severe asthma presents to your casualty department. How would you make a clinical assessment of the severity of the attack? (50%) What are the indications for mechanical ventilation? (25%) What strategies would you employ to ventilate this patient and why? (25%)

Clinical assessment would include

1. Brief history from patient/relatives/paramedics or other doctors attending the patient to include:
   - Speed of onset
   - Previous treatment
   - Previous attacks, hospitalisations and any need for mechanical ventilation.
2. Physical examination
   - Look for signs of acute severe asthma which include inability to talk or complete sentences, diffuse expiratory wheeze, tachycardia >110 beats/min, respiratory rate >25 breaths/min
   - More ominous signs of life-threatening asthma include a silent chest, confusion, exhaustion, cyanosis and bradycardia.

Investigations

- Peak expiratory flow rate (PEFR) of <33% of predicted is a sign of life-threatening asthma
- CXR to exclude pneumothorax
- Arterial blood gas measurement including serial measurement. Normally will show mild hypoxaemia with hypocapnia; worsening hypoxaemia with normocapnia or hypercapnia are very ominous signs.

Indications for mechanical ventilation

- Respiratory arrest
- Reduced level of consciousness or coma
- Exhaustion
- Increasing hypoxaemia or acidosis despite maximal medical therapies.

Strategies for mechanical ventilation

There are many changes in lung physiology of acute asthma which make mechanical ventilation hazardous.

- Airflow obstruction, leading to high inflation pressures, barotrauma and a risk of pneumothorax.

- Lung units will have variably increased time constants. Long inspiratory times may be necessary to provide adequate time for gas exchange as well as long expiratory times to allow deflation and avoid auto PEEP.
- Overinflation reduces venous return, increases pulmonary vascular resistance and compresses the heart. This will have the effect of impairing cardiac output.

In light of these problems strategies to ventilate the patient would include:
- Low respiratory rate
- Low tidal volumes, either volume-controlled or pressure-controlled, though if pressure-controlled care must be taken that an adequate volume is being delivered
- Limiting airway pressures
- Altered inspiratory:expiratory ratio with a prolonged expiratory time
- Permissive hypercapnia
- Prolonged muscle paralysis and sedation with bronchodilating drugs such as ketamine may be necessary if the bronchospasm is difficult to reverse.

Ref: Webb A R, Shapiro M, Singer M, Suter P. *Oxford textbook of critical care*. Oxford: Oxford University Press, 1999 pp 90–95.

4. What is latex allergy? (30%) Who is at risk of developing latex allergy? (20%) How would you manage a 55-year-old with latex allergy for a check cystoscopy? (50%)

There are many different latex proteins that may be implicated in the allergic response to latex as well as the chemicals used in the manufacturing process.

There are two types of allergic reaction:
- Type IV delayed hypersensitivity reaction which is T cell mediated. This is a reaction to the chemical accelerators, antioxidants or stabilisers used in the manufacturing process producing a localised contact dermatitis.
- Type I immediate hypersensitivity reaction to the latex proteins. It is IgE mediated in a previously sensitised individual and presents as anaphylaxis, classically 30–60 min after the start of exposure.

High-risk groups
This includes people who are repeatedly exposed to latex such as:

- Health care workers
- Patients undergoing repeated medical or surgical procedures, particularly chronic bladder catheterisation.
- Patients with a strong history of atopy (they may show cross reactivity with certain foods such as banana or avocado)
- The prevalence in individuals with spina bifida may be as high as 60% due to reason two above.

Management

The aim of management is to avoid exposure to the allergen as well as to maintain a high index of suspicion in the high-risk groups.

- As an elective case, there is time to prepare both the ward and theatre environment for the case.
- Patient should be nursed in a side room with visible signs to alert health care workers.
- The patient should be first on the theatre list in a theatre which has been emptied of latex equipment and unoccupied for the preceding 2 h.
- Pre-medication may be considered, though it is of no proven benefit, with H_1, H_2 blockade and hydrocortisone for 24 h prior and 12 h post procedure.
- Intra-operatively a standard anaesthetic is administered ensuring that only equipment which is free from latex is used; this may include some types of syringes, blood pressure cuffs and the mattress of the operating table.
- Postoperatively the patient should remain in the recovery area for up to 30 min to allow time for any presentation after a short procedure.

Ref: Farley C A, Jones H M. Latex allergy. *Br J Anaesth CEPD Rev* 2002; **2(1)**:20–23.

5. A 5-year-old boy is brought into the emergency room after being rescued from a pond. The monitor shows fine ventricular fibrillation. Describe your resuscitation including relevant drugs, with doses, and equipment sizes.

A 5-year-old chid will weigh approximately 18 kg [(age + 4)×2] and require an endotracheal tube of internal diameter 5.0 mm [(age/4)+4]. Resuscitation should follow the guidelines produced by the Resuscitation Council (UK) 2006.

Assuming Basic Life Support (BLS) is ongoing on arrival in the emergency room, this should be stopped momentarily for an assessment of the airway (opened with a jaw thrust, keeping the cervical spine in the neutral position in case of concomitant spinal injury). Then breathing is assessed, looking listening and feeling for 10 s whilst also feeling for a carotid pulse. Once cardiorespiratory arrest is confirmed the cardiac arrest team should be called if they are not already present.

Once cardiorespiratory arrest is confirmed oxygenate the child with high-concentration oxygen initially with a bag-valve-mask followed by intubation using a 5.0 uncuffed endotracheal tube. Give 2 ventilations followed by 15 chest compressions at a rate of 100/min using the heel of one hand over the lower third of the sternum. Once the child is intubated the compressions and ventilations should continue asynchronously, compressions at 100/min and ventilations at 10/min.

Attach the cardiac monitor and confirm the rhythm. The treatment for fine ventricular fibrillation (VF) is defibrillation at 70 J (4 J/kg) after ensuring the victim has been thoroughly dried. After the shock resume chest compressions and ventilations for 2 min, before reassessing rhythm.

IV or if that fails intra-osseous (IO) access should be obtained and adrenaline 180 μg (10 μg/kg) given, which is repeated every 3–5 min during resuscitation.

A low reading rectal thermometer should be inserted to check the victim's core temperature. If severely hypothermic <30°C withhold repeated doses of adrenaline and once above 30°C give doses every 6–10 min. Defibrillation will be ineffective in the hypothermic subject; after three shocks withhold further shocks until the core temperature is above 30°C.

During this time BLS is ongoing and the subject should be actively re-warmed. Re- warming measures include removing any wet clothing, using forced air warming blankets, giving warmed IV fluids in aliquots of 360 ml (20 ml/kg), using warmed gases and gastric, peritoneal and bladder lavage. Cardiopulmonary by-pass can be used if available.

Other potential causes of cardiac arrest should be sought and reversed, in particular any evidence of toxin ingestion or trauma. If the subject is hypothermic resuscitation may be prolonged, CPR should continue uninterrupted unless there is a change to a perfusing rhythm with a pulse or a visible sign of life. Death cannot be confirmed until the patient has been re-warmed above 34°C or until all attempts to raise the temperature have failed.

Ref : *Advanced Life Support,* Resuscitation Council (UK) 2006

Advanced Paediatric Life Support 2001

6. Discuss the principles of management of a 35-year-old patient with myasthenia gravis who requires a thymectomy.

Myasthenia gravis is a rare disease characterised by fatigable muscle weakness resulting from a failure of neuromuscular transmission. In 10% of patients a thymoma is present and thymectomy is commonly performed.

Anaesthetic considerations

- There may be associated autoimmune disorders such as thyroid, collagen vascular or rheumatoid arthritis which will influence the anaesthetic.
- Preoperative evaluation of respiratory function is vital. Forced vital capacity (FVC) is used as a marker of respiratory muscle capacity. Muscle weakness will impair coughing and clearing secretions both pre and post operatively. Bulbar muscle weakness will increase the possibility of aspiration and infection preoperatively and may necessitate a nasogastric tube.
- Preoperative therapy may include high-dose steroids or immunosuppression and occasionally plasmapheresis. Anticholinesterases are the mainstay of treatment, and they should be reduced by ~20% preoperatively or omitted on the day of surgery.
- Intraoperative intubation is required and can be achieved using a propofol/opiate technique or, if using muscle paralysis, a non-depolarising blocker at a dose of 10% normal. Monitoring of neuromuscular transmission is essential and spontaneous return of neuromuscular function is used to avoid confusion with reversal agents. These patients are relatively resistant to suxamethonium and if it is necessary to perform a rapid sequence induction due to the bulbar weakness, a dose of 2 mg/kg is used.
- A nasogastric tube, if not already in situ, should be inserted to allow postoperative anticholinesterase therapy to be administered, usually in a reduced dose.
- Large-bore IV access should be inserted in a pedal vein to ensure systemic delivery of drugs in the event of the superior vena cava being injured during the operation.
- Careful monitoring of IV fluid replacement and electrolytes intraoperatively is required, as hypovolaemia, hypokalaemia and hypothermia will all exacerbate muscle weakness.
- Postoperatively, management in a high dependency unit is optimal. A few patients may need prolonged ventilation but most can be extubated, with aggressive physiotherapy, oxygen and attention to

pain relief. Some may require non-invasive ventilatory support whilst anticholinesterases are re-introduced.

7. What are the specific problems associated with anaesthesia for elective surgery in the patient with dialysis-dependent renal failure.

Patients with chronic renal failure have multiple co-morbidities which will impact on anaesthesia. They also have altered drug handling due to chronic uraemia and acidosis.

Co-morbidities include:

1. Diseases that have caused the renal failure, eg diabetes mellitus or collagen vascular diseases.
2. Diseases that have resulted from the renal failure:
   - *Anaemia*: commonly normochromic normocytic due to reduced erythropoietin and chronic disease. There may also be iron deficiency due to losses from haemodialysis or peptic ulceration. It is often treated with recombinant erythropoietin injections. Patients may require preoperative transfusion although anaemia is well tolerated due to shift of the oxyhaemoglobin dissociation curve by raised 2,3-DPG and acidosis.
   - *Clotting disorders* due to impaired platelet function from uraemia. The risks and benefits of neuroaxial blockade must be carefully assessed.
   - *Cardiovascular disease* is common. Hypertension occurs either primarily or secondary to the renal failure and is present in up to 80% of patients. There may be exaggerated responses to induction and laryngoscopy.
     Ischaemic heart disease, which may be silent, congestive cardiac failure and cardiomyopathy are all common. Pericarditis may occur due to uraemia.
     Vascular access may be difficult due to multiple previous catheters and or A–V shunts. Any functioning shunts should be kept warm, padded and avoiding any blood pressure cuffs.
   - *Respiratory disease*. Pulmonary oedema may be present from fluid overload or from cardiac origin. Fibrosis can occur due to medical conditions or therapies.
   - *Autonomic neuropathy* is common in diabetics
   - *Increased acid* production and delayed gastric emptying both predispose to reflux and aspiration. A rapid sequence induction may be required and antacids are often prescribed as pre-medication.

3. Other consequences of renal failure to consider
   - Calcium may be high or low; hypomagnesaemia will potentiate neuromuscular blockade. Hyperkalaemia is common, so the potassium level should be known preoperatively and suxamethonium should be avoided if possible.
   - The patient's 'ideal weight' should be known together with normal urine output, diuretic therapy and most recent dialysis, with the post dialysis [K^+] level and haemoglobin concentration.
   - The timing of dialysis prior to surgery. If immediately prior to surgery, patients are commonly fluid depleted and may need fluid replacement prior to induction.
   - Central venous pressure monitoring will be helpful to guide fluid replacement intra- and post-operatively and continuous cardiac output monitoring will be helpful in those with cardiac disease or those with large fluid shifts having major surgery.
   - Pharmacokinetics and dynamics are altered. Reduced protein binding means that lower doses of drugs such as benzodiazepines or barbiturates are needed. Renally excreted drugs or metabolites will accumulate, eg morphine-6-glucuronide, therefore reduced doses are needed. Atracurium is the muscle relaxant of choice as it is degraded rather than renally excreted.
   - HDU or ITU may be required postoperatively with attention to fluid balance and the timing of postoperative dialysis.

Ref: Holland D E, Old S. Anaesthesia for patients with impaired renal function. *Curr Anaesth Crit Care* 1992; **3**:140–145.

8. Describe the principles involved in the pulse oximetry (50%). What are its limitations in clinical practice? (50%)

Principles

- Differential absorption of red and infra-red light by oxygenated and deoxygenated haemoglobin.
- At 660 nm oxyhaemoglobin absorbs less light than deoxyhaemoglobin and this is reversed at 940 nm. The isosbestic point, ie where the two absorption coefficients are identical, is 800 nm.
- The pulse oximeter uses two light-emitting diodes which produce pulses of red (660 nm) and infra-red (940 nm) light. The light is shone through the tissue and sensed by a photocell on the other side of the electrode.

- The output is electronically processed to produce a ratio of the absorption of the two light wavelengths. This is then compared to an algorithm to calculate the % oxygenated haemoglobin.

Errors and limitations

- Calibration is only accurate within the range 70%–100%, increasingly inaccurate at lower arterial blood oxygen saturation (SpO_2).
- Bright direct sunlight will interfere with use.
- Hypoperfusion of tissue from hypothermia, low cardiac output or vasoconstriction will give inaccurate results.
- Inaccurate results from movement artefact or electrical interference (not a major problem).
- Absorption of infra-red light by other substances, eg nail varnish or bilirubin, will give an abnormally low reading. Systemic dyes such as methylene blue will also interfere with red light absorption.
- Absorption by abnormal haemoglobins
  - High concentrations of carboxyhaemoglobin, eg following smoke inhalation, will give an abnormally high reading.
  - High levels of methaemoglobin in blood, eg following nitric oxide therapy, will give a reading usually around 85%.
- The oximeter measures the % of oxygenated haemoglobin. It does not measure tissue oxygenation, which may be inadequate with a high SpO_2 if there is severe anaemia. Although it gives information on oxygenation of the blood it gives no information on the adequacy of ventilation.

9. Describe the nerve supply to the foot. (40%) How would you perform an ankle block? (60%)

There are five nerves which supply the foot:

1. **The saphenous nerve**
   A terminal branch of the femoral nerve, it supplies sensation to the medial border of the foot and ankle. At the ankle it lies immediately anterior to the medial malleolus where it lies close to the long saphenous vein.
2. **Sural nerve**
   A branch of the tibial nerve. It enters the foot lying superficially behind the lateral malleolus to supply sensation to the 5th toe and lateral border of the foot.

3. **Posterior tibial nerve**
   A branch of the sciatic nerve. It lies behind the medial malleolus where it is posterior to the posterior tibial artery. It supplies sensation to the plantar surface of the foot.
4. **Deep peroneal nerve**
   Enters the foot beneath the extensor retinaculum between the tendons of extensor hallucis and extensor digitorum longus. It supplies sensation to a small area between the 1st and 2nd toes on the dorsum of the foot.
5. **Superficial peroneal nerve**
   A branch of the common peroneal nerve, it runs superficially over the dorsum of the ankle between the medial and lateral malleoli where it divides into multiple terminal branches. It supplies sensation to much of the dorsum of the foot except that supplied by the deep peroneal and sural nerves.

Ankle block

- Check there are no absolute or relative contraindications to the nerve block such as local infection, coagulopathy or concurrent neurological disease.
- Obtain informed consent from the patient including significant risks which include failure, infection, intravascular injection and neurological damage.
- Prepare the equipment, including a short bevelled 23-G needle, local anaesthetic solution, intravenous access and full resuscitation equipment.
- If performed awake explain the need for four injections:
  1. Saphenous nerve blocked immediately anterior to the medial malleolus.
  2. Superficial peroneal and sural nerves blocked by superficial infiltration over the dorsum of the ankle between the medial and lateral malleoli.
  3. Deep peroneal nerve blocked by injection between the tendons of tibialis anterior and extensor hallucis longus under the extensor retinaculum adjacent to the dorsalis pedis artery.
  4. Tibial nerve blocked by injecting anterolaterally to the posterior tibial artery posterior to the medial malleolus.

10. Summarise the peri-operative management of a 55-year-old with a body mass index of 38 kg·m^{-2} who requires a laparoscopic cholecystectomy.

A body mass index [weight (kg)/height (m)^2] of 38 kg·m^{-2} classifies this subject as morbidly obese. This poses many problems for the anaesthetist.

Preoperatively

- A thorough cardiovascular assessment is essential. Hypertension and ischaemic heart disease are both common co-morbidities and should be investigated and treated. Glucose intolerance is also common.
- The increased blood volume and cardiac output leads to cardiomegaly, left ventricular hypertrophy and the potential for left ventricular failure.
- Obesity is a significant risk factor for venous thromboembolism. Thromboembolic deterrent stockings and low-molecular-weight heparin should be started preoperatively and continued until discharge.
- The airway should be assessed, as difficulty with intubation is common; mask ventilation may also be challenging. There is increased oxygen consumption and carbon dioxide production as well as an increased work of breathing due to reduced chest wall and lung compliance.
- Obstructive sleep apnoea is common, and untreated may lead to pulmonary hypertension, right ventricular hypertrophy and right ventricular failure.
- Increased acidity and volume of gastric contents together with a high incidence of hiatus hernia predispose to acid reflux and aspiration. A rapid sequence induction or awake fibre optic intubation may be necessary together with pre medication with antacids and prokinetics.

Intraoperatively

- Venous access is difficult and may necessitate central venous access, and/or the use of ultrasound to locate veins.
- Monitoring may be difficult, particularly the use of non-invasive blood pressure cuffs, and invasive arterial pressure monitoring will overcome this.
- Transferring, positioning and surgical access are all difficult.
- The reduced compliance and functional residual capacity both predispose to shunt, atelectasis and hypoxia. Intubation and ventilation will be required, the addition of PEEP will improve

oxygenation, but the reduced compliance will cause high airway pressures, which will be worsened by the pneumoperitoneum.
- Cardiac output may be severely compromised by the pneumoperitoneum and occasionally conversion to an open operation may be necessary.
- Drug dosages should be calculated on lean body mass; fat-soluble anaesthetic agents will accumulate therefore the least soluble agents should be used.

Postoperatively
- Patient should be extubated awake and sitting upright to reduce the work of breathing and improve pulmonary compliance.
- A high dependency environment is essential if there is obstructive sleep apnoea and is desirable for oxygen therapy and non-invasive ventilatory support.
- Good analgesia to allow coughing, physiotherapy and early mobilisation.

Ref: Adams J P and Murphy P G. Obesity in anaesthesia and intensive care. *Br J Anaesth* 2000; **85**: 91–108.

11. How may homologous blood transfusion be minimised peri-operatively?

An integrated approach involving pre-, intra- and post-operative strategies.

Preoperatively
- Diagnosis, investigation and treatment of anaemia preoperatively including liaison with haematologists.
- Stop drugs which will interfere with the coagulation process preoperatively if feasible, such as aspirin, clopidogrel and non-steroidal anti-inflammatory drugs.
- Pre-donation. Up to 5 units of blood may be donated over a 5-week period, and can be combined with iron and erythropoietin to boost haemoglobin production.

Intra-operatively
- Acute normovolaemic haemodilution, whereby whole blood is withdrawn at the start of the operation and replaced by a combination of colloid and crystalloid. Intraoperative blood loss has a lower haematocrit thus reducing absolute haemoglobin loss; once haemostasis is achieved the patient's whole blood is returned.

- Use of cell salvage, not suitable for oncology patients. Red cells are washed and reinfused, without platelets or clotting factors. Suitable in situations where blood loss exceeds ~1000 ml.
- Surgical techniques. Use of lasers and harmonic scalpels can reduce surgical bleeding.
- Pharmacological. Use of vasoconstrictors in situations such as plastic surgery, or anti-fibrinolytics such as tranexamic acid or aprotinin in cardiac, liver or orthopaedic surgery. There may be a risk of pro-coagulation in some circumstances, eg graft occlusion post cardiac by-pass surgery.

Postoperatively

- Postoperative cell salvage, suitable in situations where the majority of blood loss occurs in the postoperative period such as knee arthroplasty. Specialised drains allow collection, filtration and return of the blood to the patient.
- Acceptance of a lower level of haemoglobin; in a fit individual no transfusion is required when the haemoglobin is 7 g/dl or above, though 10 g/dl may be required in those with cardiorespiratory disease.
- Prescription of iron supplements postoperatively.

Ref: The Association of Anaesthetists of Great Britain and Ireland. *Blood transfusion and the anaesthetist*. 2005. London: The Association of Anaesthetists of Great Britain and Ireland.

12. What are the options for pain relief following a thoracotomy? (40%) What are the advantages and disadvantages of each? (60%)

Acute post thoracotomy pain is aggravated by the constant movement of breathing and is thus widely regarded as being one of the most painful surgical procedures. However, aggressive physiotherapy is essential to prevent atelectasis, secretion retention and ventilatory failure and this can only be achieved with optimal analgesia.

Analgesic options can be broadly divided into two categories, though in practice a mixture of the two is commonly used to provide balanced multi-modal analgesia.

Systemic

- *Parenteral opioid infusions*
  Patient-controlled analgesia (PCA) with a background infusion is commonly used. Sedation, respiratory depression, nausea and

vomiting and cough suppression are all undesirable side-effects. Pain relief may be inadequate when used alone. Nursing in a high dependency area is desirable. It is easy to institute and non-invasive.

- *Other systemic analgesics*
  Paracetamol is commonly prescribed for its morphine-sparing properties though non-steroidal anti-inflammatories are often withheld in the acute phase for fear of renal toxicity in potentially dehydrated patients in the immediate postoperative period.

Regional

- *Epidural analgesia*
  Catheter usually sited at the mid point of the dermatomal distribution of the skin incision to minimise the amount of local anaesthetic/opioid mixture required and therefore minimise unwanted effects. These include motor and sympathetic blockade, leading to impaired cough and hypotension. Placement may be technically challenging and there is a 15% failure rate. It is an invasive procedure and complications of catheter placement are serious, including spinal cord compression or damage and epidural abscess.
  Benefits of this technique include superior analgesia compared to parenteral opioids with less sedation and possibly improved respiratory function.
- *Intrathecal opioids*
  Usually administered as a single dose of morphine into the lumbar CSF. The morphine migrates to the thoracic region, however it may spread further rostrally leading to severe respiratory depression which occurs in up to 25% of patients. A catheter is not left in situ therefore repeated doses cannot be given, however it carries all the risks of accessing the CSF including headache, infection and neurological damage.
- *Paravertebral nerve block*
  A catheter is introduced either using loss of resistance or under direct vision by the surgeon. The advantages are of unilateral sympathetic and motor block and therefore less hypotension and better preserved respiratory function. Neurological damage, infection and CSF tap are potential complications.
- *Intercostal nerve block*
  Quick and simple to perform, usually performed as single injections and therefore short acting. Multiple catheters can be sited but are generally time consuming and too complicated to be used routinely.

Side-effects include bleeding and nerve damage though these are uncommon.

- *Inter-pleural analgesia*
  Local anaesthetic is injected between the visceral and parietal pleura either as a single injection or as an infusion. Results are variable as the local anaesthetic solution tends to pool in dependent areas and be lost through chest drains.

Ref: Hughes R. Pain control for thoracotomy. *Br J Anaesth CEPD* 2005; **5** (No 2): 56–60.

Multiple Choice Question Paper 4 Answers

1 Magnetic resonance imaging **Answers: B D**

Atom nuclei with unpaired protons or neutrons are aligned in the field (eg hydrogen). Blood is dark in T_1-weighted scans, bright in T_2-weighted scans. MRI is better than CT at visualising inside bony structures, such as the posterior fossa, the pelvis, and the spinal canal. Images can be reconstructed in any plane.

2 Infrared spectrophotometry can be used to measure the following **Answers: B D E**

Infrared radiation is absorbed by covalent bonds between two different atoms in a molecule. Molecules have peaks of absorption at characteristic frequencies.

3 The Clarke oxygen electrode **Answers: A C D E**

Unlike the fuel cell whose reaction generates its own power, the Clarke electrode requires a battery power source. It has a silver/silver anode and a platinum cathode (the fuel cell has a lead anode). Reduction of other things at the cathode, such as nitrous oxide or halothane, can cause inaccuracies, and so a specific semi-permeable membrane is used.

4 The reading of the pulse oximeter can be unreliable in the following circumstances **Answers: A E**

Pulse oximeters commonly sample at two wavelengths: 660 nm for deoxyhaemoglobin and 940 nm for oxyhaemoglobin. Carboxyhaemoglobin has low absorbance at 660 nm but high absorbance at 940 nm, causing an overestimation of oxygen saturation. Fetal and sickle cell haemoglobin have similar absorbance spectra to adult haemoglobin, and so have no effect on oximetry. There is a linear trend to underestimate saturations with increasing anaemia, although polycythaemia has no effect.

5 The Tec6 desflurane vaporiser **Answers: C E**

Desflurane has a boiling point of 23°C, and a high saturated vapour pressure (SVP) of 88 kPa at 20°C, so would be constantly on the boil in a normal vaporiser, risking overdose. It is heated to 39°C because of the high SVP to enable consistency in vapour pressure. An internal pressure transducer compares the vapour pressure with the fresh gas flow pressure, adjusting the rate of release of vapour to achieve the dialled up concentration. It is colour-coded blue. All plenum vaporisers have high internal resistance, making them unsuitable to be used within the circuit.

6 Cardiorespiratory exercise (CPX) testing **Answers: A C D E**

CPX testing is an integrated method of evaluating oxygen uptake in the lungs, and its delivery to the tissues by the cardiovascular system. Subjects exercise against a continuously increasing resistance, either on an exercise bike or with a hand crank. The system measures the heart and respiratory rate, the tidal volume, and the composition of inspired and expired gases. A continuous 12-lead ECG is also performed. A plot of VCO_2 vs VO_2 suddenly changes gradient at the point when the increase in production of CO_2 outstrips the increase in consumption of O_2, this extra CO_2 being produced by anaerobic respiration (the anaerobic threshold). An AT of <11 ml/min per kg has been shown to be associated with worse perioperative mortality in preliminary studies.
http://www.cpxtesting.com

7 Concerning fetal monitoring during labour **Answers: A B C**

Loss of baseline variability may reflect a fetus who is sleeping, the effects of drugs (eg diazepam, diamorphine) or fetal hypoxia. Early decelerations coincide with uterine contraction and reflect fetal vagal tone as the head is squashed. Late decelerations (30 s after peak contraction) reflect hypoxia. The normal fetal scalp pH is 7.3–7.4 (down to 7.15 during second stage); levels <7.2, if not in the second stage, require immediate delivery.

8 The oesophageal Doppler **Answers: A D E**

Oesophageal Doppler probes can be inserted orally or nasally. The velocity of blood in the descending aorta is estimated continuously from the shift in frequency (not phase) between transmitted and reflected ultrasound. The FTc is a number which reflects ejection time, corrected for heart rate, and is related to left ventricular end-diastolic volume.

9 BIS monitor **Answers: A B C**

BIS monitors the frontotemporal EEG trace and processes the raw data to generate a number between 0 and 100, 0 being no cortical activity and 100 being normal cortical activity. The score at which subjects stop responding shows variation, depending on the stimulus and the individual, but the consensus is that the probability of recall is very low if the BIS is kept <60. BIS shows a dose-dependent response for the volatile anaesthetic agents (although N_2O is more complex), and the intravenous agents including propofol and midazolam. Ketamine however causes EEG activation, complicating the interpretation. In practice the BIS monitor helps anaesthetists find the balance of analgesia and anaesthesia required, and usually results in less anaesthetic being given.

10 Intracranial pressure monitoring **Answers: A B C**

Intracranial pressure monitoring can be extradural with a fibre optic probe (having the lowest infection rates); a subarachnoid screw (easy to place); via a ventricular drain (highest infection risk); and intracerebral (in the tissue itself). The basic waveform has spikes corresponding to the pulsation of large blood vessels. When ventilated the CVP rises in inspiration, causing a rise in intracranial pressure. A waves (amplitude 50–100 mmHg, lasting 5–20 min) are associated with severely reduced intracranial compliance.

11 Fixed cardiac output state **Answers: A B D E**

In both aortic stenosis and hypertrophic obstructive cardiomyopathy (HOCM), there is obstruction to the outflow from the left ventricle either at the level of the valve or sub-valvular. This results in a fixed, low cardiac output state.

In mitral stenosis there is also a fixed low cardiac output state as there is obstruction to the passage of blood from the left atrium to the left ventricle through the mitral valve.

In constrictive pericarditis the ventricles cannot relax fully in diastole so that ventricular filling is inadequate and the cardiac output is therefore low and also fixed.

In patent ductus arteriosus (PDA), by contrast, there is a hyperdynamic circulation with a collapsing pulse and a high cardiac output as there is a connection between the aorta and the pulmonary artery.

12 Ulcerative colitis **Answers: A B C D**

Ulcerative colitis is an inflammatory condition of the colon. It is often accompanied by liver disease ranging from ascending cholangitis to cirrhosis. In long-standing disease there is a significant risk of malignant change. Patients may show clubbing of the fingers. Treatment may involve the use of corticosteroids.

13 Obstructive jaundice **Answers: B C E**

In obstructive jaundice the patient may complain of pale stools and dark urine. This is because there is no stercobilin in the stools and an elevated amount of conjugated bilirubin in the urine. Because there is obstruction to the passage of bile into the gut there is reduced vitamin K absorption and a resultant coagulopathy. In addition lack of bile salts leads to defective gut absorption of the other fat-soluble vitamins (A, D, E) and of fat itself, leading to steatorrhoea. The stools have a high faecal fat content and therefore tend to float.

Classically, in obstructive jaundice, the alkaline phosphatase and gamma-glutamyl transpeptidase are elevated, compared with an elevated aspartate transaminase and alanine aminotransferase in jaundice from hepatocellular damage.

14 Reticulocytosis **Answers: C E**

A raised reticulocyte count indicates haemolysis. A reticulocytosis will occur once iron deficiency or megaloblastic anaemia is treated. Sickle cell disease, but not the trait, leads to a haemolytic state. Congenital spherocytosis is a hereditary haemolytic disorder.

15 Mitral stenosis **Answers: A B D E**

Mitral stenosis is associated with a loud first heart sound, an opening snap and a low-pitched rumbling mid-diastolic murmur heard best at the apex with the patient lying in the left lateral position. Atrial fibrillation is common in mitral valve disease. The patient often has a malar flush. The apex beat is tapping in quality, but is not displaced.

16 Vomiting **Answers: A B E**

Vomiting leads to loss of HCl from the stomach, leading to a metabolic alkalosis. The resulting dehydration causes a raised blood urea. The kidney attempts to compensate by conserving hydrogen ions in exchange for potassium, hence the alkaline urine and low plasma potassium. Hyperkalaemia in itself does not cause vomiting.

17 Crohn's disease **Answers: A B C E**

Crohn's is a granulomatous condition affecting the bowel. It is associated with fistulae and perianal sepsis. Arthritis, uveitis and skin rashes may occur. Lymphoma is associated with coeliac disease.

18 Glycosuria **Answers: A B E**

Glycosuria occurs commonly in pregnancy. It is found in subarachnoid haemorrhage and phaeochromocytoma due to the high levels of circulating catecholamines. Hypopituitarism and partial gastrectomy are causes of hypoglycaemia.

19 Spironolactone therapy **Answers: B D**

Spironolactone is a potassium-sparing diuretic and an antagonist of aldosterone. It thus causes hyperkalaemia and hyponatraemia. The thiazide diuretics cause hyponatraemia, hyperuricaemia, glucose intolerance, hypokalaemia and metabolic alkalosis.

20 Megaloblastic anaemia **Answers: B C D E**

Megaloblastic anaemia may be caused by deficiency of vitamin B_{12} or folic acid. The red cells of the blood are macrocytic with an elevated mean corpuscular volume (MCV). Vitamin B_{12} deficiency is most often due to autoimmune destruction of gastric parietal cells, so-called Addisonian pernicious anaemia (PA). B_{12} is normally bound by intrinsic factor (IF), produced by gastric parietal cells. The B_{12} + IF complex is then absorbed in the terminal ileum. Thus disease or surgical resection of the stomach or terminal ileum may result in megaloblastic anaemia. As gastric parietal cells produce acid as well as IF achlorhydria is a feature of PA. Gastric cancer is an association of PA. Nitrous oxide can cause megaloblastic anaemia with a normal serum B_{12}.

Exposure of >6 h can cause this effect by inhibition of the enzyme methionine synthetase. Chronic exposure to nitrous oxide may, rarely, lead to a neurological picture similar to the peripheral neuropathy and sub-acute combined degeneration of the cord seen in vitamin B_{12} deficiency. Megaloblastosis may be caused by dietary deficiency of folic acid or may be due to antifolate drugs such as trimethoprim, phenytoin or methotrexate. Other causes of macrocytosis include hypothyroidism, alcohol and liver disease.

21 Prothrombin time **Answer: D**

The prothrombin time is a test of the extrinsic pathway of the clotting cascade and is therefore affected by changes in factor 7 or the common pathway. Haemophilia leads to a prolongation of the APTT, as does von Willebrand's disease. In addition the bleeding time is prolonged in von Willebrand's disease. Scurvy, deficiency of vitamin C, leads to defective collagen synthesis. The weak collagen in the vascular connective tissue leads to a prolonged bleeding time. In jaundiced patients there is a deficiency of the vitamin-K-dependent clotting factors (2, 7, 9 and 10) leading to a prolongation of both the PT and APTT. Thrombocytopenic purpura is due to immune destruction of platelets and only the bleeding time is prolonged.

22 Cataract is caused by **Answers: A B C D**

Cataract is the commonest cause of blindness in the world. It affects 75% of over 65s. The commonest cause in Britain is ageing, followed by diabetes. Other causes include galactosaemia, hypocalcaemia, intrauterine rubella or toxoplasmosis, trauma, electric shock, irradiation and genetic (such as myotonia). Thyrotoxicosis is a cause of glaucoma.

23 The generic pacemaker code **Answers: A B E**

Position 1 is the chamber paced, 2 the chamber sensed and 3 the response. An 'I' in 3 means the response is inhibited if there is a spontaneous ventricular complex sensed. Position 4 defines the programmability of rate modulation and 5 the functions available for tachycardia.

24 Pneumothorax **Answers: A B C E**

The causes can be grouped to three anatomic mechanisms:

- Intrapulmonary rupture – high pressures during IPPV, severe cough, spontaneous

- Visceral pleura injury – lung biopsy, ruptured bulla, fractured rib, central line insertion
- Parietal pleura injury – open chest wound, oesophageal perforation, post tracheostomy or thyroidectomy.

It is best diagnosed (if there are no signs of tension) by an erect CXR in expiration. N_2O will increase the size of a pneumothorax as it is more soluble than N_2, so should not be used unless a chest drain is in place.

25 Oesophageal atresia **Answers: C E**

85% of these babies also have tracheo-oesophageal fistula. Unlike diaphragmatic hernia face mask ventilation is not contraindicated, but care must be taken not to over inflate the stomach. It can present with cough, airway obstruction, excessive secretions, abdominal distension and recurrent pneumonia. Contrast should be avoided as it may get into the lung. Diagnosis is by seeing a coiled NG tube in the oesophagus on CXR or by endoscopy.

26 The thalassaemias **Answers: B D**

The thalassaemias are genetic diseases of unbalanced haemoglobin synthesis. Adult haemoglobin is composed of two α chains and two β chains (HbA = $\alpha_2\beta_2$). Normally we have four sets of α genes and two sets of β genes. HbF is $\alpha_2\gamma_2$, and persists in β thalassaemia where there is a deficiency in production of β chains. In the nomenclature $^+$ means reduced production and ^{0} means no production. In α/α^+ three of the four α genes are working, so the disease is very mild or 'silent'. In β/β^+ there is reduced production by one of the two β genes but only mild anaemia (Hb usually >9 g/dl) and splenomegaly is rare. The more severe diseases require repeated transfusions, aiming for an Hb >9 g/dl. Iron overload becomes a problem, causing cardiac and liver disease and endocrine failure (diabetes mellitus). Desferrioxamine, an iron chelator, provides some protection.

27 Autonomic neuropathy **Answers: A B C D E**

It results in postural hypotension, cardiac conduction defects, and bladder and gut dysfunction. It can be caused by diabetes, amyloidosis, autoimmune diseases, porphyria, Guillain-Barré and CNS problems such as infection, CVA and Shy–Drager syndrome.

28 Developmental milestones **Answers: A C**

Three-month-old babies should be able to smile, at least some of the time. Most walk by the age of 18 months. By 2½ a mother should understand her child's speech most of the time, the child should understand simple instructions like 'get your shoes' and can already say things like 'I want cake'. By 3½ children should have a vocabulary of 1000 words. Delays may mean unrecognised deafness, cognitive impairment or deprivation.

29 Amphotericin B **Answers: A C E**

Amphoteracin B is used to treat invasive aspergillosis (steroids are the treatment in allergic aspergillosis). It commonly causes nephrotoxicity and is given over 24 h to try to reduce the risks of anaphylaxis, arrhythmias, seizures and other unpleasant side-effects. Ambisome, liposomal amphotericin, has a much better side-effect profile.

30 Acute cholecystitis **Answers: A B D E**

Murphy's sign – palpate the right upper quadrant (RUQ) with two fingers, ask patient to breathe in, pain arrests inspiration as inflamed gall bladder meets fingers (it is only positive if it is negative in the LUQ). If the stone moves to the common bile duct it may cause obstructive jaundice. Ultrasound may show an inflamed gall bladder. Treatment can involve cholecystectomy within 48 h in suitable patients, or otherwise after 3 months.

31 Specific gravity of urine **Answers: A B D**

Diabetes insipidus (which may occur with lithium toxicity) leads to the production of large amounts of dilute urine, as either the renal tubules fail to respond to ADH or the posterior pituitary fails to produce ADH.

In diabetes mellitus the glucose in the urine raises its specific gravity. In intestinal obstruction the resulting dehydration causes oliguria and the production of small amounts of concentrated urine, while in acute tubular necrosis small amounts of poor quality urine are produced.

32 Cardiac tamponade **Answers: A B C**

Cardiac tamponade is associated with an elevated JVP and a reduced cardiac output. The radial pulse is weak and becomes even weaker on inspiration, so-called pulsus paradoxus. It may be differentiated from CCF as it is associated with a small heart on CXR, little or no pulmonary oedema, and hepatomegaly and ascites. It requires pericardiocentesis or surgery.

33 Intravenous propranolol **Answers: C D**

Propranolol is a non-selective beta-blocking drug. It may cause bronchoconstriction and is both negatively inotropic and chronotropic. In patients receiving verapamil, beta blockers can cause profound hypotension and bradycardia. Although beta blockers mask the response to hypoglycaemia they do not cause hyperglycaemia. Lignocaine is the agent of choice for the treatment of ventricular ectopic beats post myocardial infarction.

34 Concerning the 2005 Resuscitation Council guidelines on adult defibrillation **Answers: B D**

When using a monophasic defibrillator all shocks should be delivered at 360 J. Biphasic defibrillators are able to compensate for variations in bioimpedance, the minimum energy level for defibrillation is 150 J. No particular biphasic waveform has been shown to be superior.

35 Following massive blood transfusion **Answer: C**

It is uncommon for the citric acid anticoagulant to cause an acidosis, citrate is metabolised in the liver to bicarbonate which may result in an alkalosis. Hypothermia and 2,3-DPG both cause a left shift in the oxyhaemoglobin dissociation curve.

36 Intrinsic PEEP **Answers: A B D E**

Dynamic hyperinflation and intrinsic PEEP occur when the duration of expiration is insufficient to allow the lungs to deflate to the relaxation volume prior to the next inspiration. This causes the inspiratory muscles to work at a mechanically disadvantageous shorter length and increases both resistive and elastic work of breathing.

37 Aspiration of gastric contents **Answers: A B E**

Aspiration occurs in up to 19% of emergency non-anaesthetic intubations compared to approximately 1 in 1000 for emergency surgery. In the ITU high-volume low-pressure endotracheal cuffs and nursing semi-recumbent both reduce the risk of aspiration. Chronic aspiration may result in nosocomial pneumonia which can be reduced by selective decontamination of the digestive tract.

38 The following initial ventilator settings are suitable for ventilating a patient with acute severe bronchospasm **Answers: All false**

The overlying principle is one of controlled hypoventilation; low tidal volume and respiratory rate and permissive hypercapnia. A prolonged expiratory time to allow alveolar emptying is balanced against allowing sufficient time for inspiration whilst limiting peak airway pressures. Although there is contention as to the optimal inspiratory flow rates, a very high flow rate of 100 l/min would result in unacceptably high peak inspiratory pressure. Although PEEP can be used to ventilate the acute asthmatic patient it is unsuitable as an **initial** ventilator setting.

39 Concerning scoring systems in ITU **Answer: C**

APACHE II uses only 12 physiological variables compared to 34 for the APACHE I and is scored using the worst score for each parameter in the first 24 h of ICU stay. It may be used for comparative audit, risk stratification and the assessment of the efficacy of ITU. The SAPS score although simplified includes scoring for three underlying chronic clinical conditions: AIDS, haematological malignancy and metastatic cancer.

40 The troponins **Answers: A B E**

Elevated troponins may reflect an area of myocardial necrosis <1.0 g and are typically elevated 4–10 h following infarction and remain raised for up to 10 days. They are also released following incomplete apoptosis as part of a non-ischaemic inflammatory process, eg sepsis. High troponin T is associated with an increased mortality in sepsis.

41 Hyperbaric oxygen therapy **Answer: C**

Vasoconstriction occurs in non-ischaemic tissue in contrast to tissues which are already ischaemic. Therefore these areas receive a greater proportion of cardiac output, this has been termed 'inverse steal'. The effects of catecholamines are enhanced and there is upregulation of insulin receptors and reduced glucagons which result in hypoglycaemia. At a partial pressure of 3 atmospheres (300 kPa) 60 ml of oxygen dissolves in 1000 ml of plasma which is sufficient to supply the metabolic demand of the whole body, therefore the mixed venous oxygen saturation will be close to 100%.

42 The following are factors increasing the risk of nosocomial infection **Answers: A B C E**

Nosocomial (caused by micro-organism acquired in hospital) infections are a major problem on ITU. The major factor is the severity of the underlying disease. Other factors can be categorised into four groups: endogenous (eg age, malnutrition, gastric pH >4, lifestyle); disease related (eg organ failure); environmental (eg hand hygiene, infection control procedures); and therapy related (eg lines, tubes, catheters, sedatives and antibiotics). In a viva you may be able to make a case for antibiotic-selective decontamination of the digestive tract possibly resulting in a reduction in infection, but that was not being asked here.

43 The following antibiotics are bacteriostatic **Answer: C**

The β-lactams (incuding penicillins, cephalosporins, and imipenem) and the glycopeptides (vancomycin and teicoplanin) attack the cell wall and are bactericidal. Drugs which disrupt nucleic acid metabolism, such as ciprofloxacin and metronidazole, are also bactericidal. Trimethoprim and the sulphonamides are antifolates and are bacteriostatic. The rest stop protein synthesis (erythromycin, fusidic acid) and are generally bacteriostatic (except gentamicin which is bactericidal). This is an example of a question where it is difficult to guess, but there was one easy mark for noticing that fluconazole, as an antifungal, did not fit.

44 Basal daily requirements for a healthy 80-kg man are **Answers: B C**

Basal requirements in mmol are: sodium 70–100; potassium 70–100; magnesium 7.5–10; calcium 5–10; phosphate 20–30.

45 Enteral nutrition for the ITU patient **Answers: A B**

Enteral nutrition reduces the risk of stress ulcers, and helps maintain intestinal barrier integrity, reducing bacterial translocation. Acute cholecystitis is a complication of TPN. It is associated (although not necessarily causally) with diarrhoea in up to 60% of patients, and in some cases is due to the osmotic load. Feeding protocols are governed by whether the feed is being absorbed and so bowel sounds are irrelevant.

46 Triage priority at a major incident **Answers: C D E**

On scene triage is a rapid, dynamic process, designed to separate those who may survive if they receive immediate or urgent treatment from those who will die soon regardless, and those who will survive if their treatment is delayed. Walking wounded are labelled delayed. No breathing despite a clear airway is labelled dead. Capillary refill >2 s (hypovolaemic shock) is potentially survivable with immediate treatment. The AVPU scale is a simple way of assessing disability. Only doctors may pronounce death.

47 Treatment of cyanide poisoning may include **Answers: A B D E**

Cyanide poisoning causes inhibition of the cytochrome oxidase system leading to histotoxic hypoxia. It may follow smoke inhalation or prolonged use of sodium nitroprusside.

48 Indications for early intubation of burn patients **Answers: A B C D E**

The feared respiratory problems are airway oedema leading to obstruction (indicated by history, voice change, stridor), lung failure (circumferential chest burns, lung damage) and histotoxic hypoxia (carboxyhaemoglobin, cyanide). Significant airway damage can be suspected from soot or burns around the nose or mouth. Inhalational injury is usually only supra-glottic, but steam may cause damage in the bronchial tree.

49 Clinical features of fulminant hepatic failure include **Answers: A B C D E**

Encephalopathy is always present in fulminant liver failure. Coagulopathy is common and is due to both a reduction in clotting factors and reduced platelet numbers and function. A hyperdynamic circulation is typical. Increased levels of circulating insulin, impaired gluconeogenesis and reduced glycogen stores frequently result in life-threatening hypoglycaemia. Sepsis is common, a normal liver clearing endotoxins from the blood, and reduced cell-mediated immunity.

50 Complications associated with total parenteral nutrition (TPN) include **Answers: A B C D E**

The complications also include problems with central venous cannulation, sepsis, lipaemia and cholestasis resulting in acute cholecystitis. Hypophosphataemia is especially marked in the refeeding syndrome.

51 Pre-eclampsia **Answers: A B**

Severe pre-eclampsia implies organ damage: blood pressure of 160/110 mmHg or greater at rest, severe proteinuria and oliguria, and central nervous system irritability, with headaches and visual problems.

Magnesium sulphate is now the anticonvulsant of choice. Magnesium is both a membrane stabiliser and a vasodilator, so improving placental blood flow. Thrombocytopenia is the most common haematological abnormality seen in severe pre-eclampsia. The HELLP syndrome (Haemolysis, Elevated Liver function tests, and Low Platelets) is a form of severe pre-eclampsia. Both the prothrombin and partial thromboplastin times are usually normal and DIC is very rare. The parturient with severe pre-eclampsia is usually advised to have a caesarean section. A regional, rather than general, anaesthesia is the preferred mode of anaesthesia as it avoids the pressor response to laryngoscopy and intubation. Although these women are often oedematous they have, nevertheless, a contracted intravascular volume. They thus require intravenous fluids in conjunction with close monitoring of urine output and central venous pressure. The aim is to avoid fluid overload and pulmonary oedema, while ensuring an adequate urine output to prevent acute renal failure.

The penicillins are active against both Gram-positive and Gram-negative organisms. It would be unusual to choose a penicillin as first-line treatment for a UTI; the commonest cause of UTI is *E. coli* for which trimethoprim is the first-choice antibiotic.

52 Contraindications to suxamethonium **Answers: A C**

There is no contraindication to the use of suxamethonium in porphyria. It is, however, a potent trigger of malignant hyperpyrexia, the other inherited condition that is of particular relevance to anaesthetists. It is contraindicated in dystrophia myotonica, where its administration may lead to such severe masseter muscle spasm as to render intubation impossible.

In acute renal failure there is hyperkalaemia. Since suxamethonium leads to a rise in serum potassium of up to 0.5–1.0 mmol/l, its administration in renal failure may precipitate cardiac arrest from ventricular fibrillation.

There is no evidence to suggest that suxamethonium is contraindicated in Creutzfeldt–Jakob disease.

Following spinal cord injury suxamethonium is indeed contraindicated, but the dangerous rise in serum potassium that its administration may cause in this situation does not occur until several days after the spinal injury.

53 Thyroid storm — Answers: A B C D E

Thyroid storm is the term given to a condition resembling acute thyrotoxicosis, occurring soon after a partial thyroidectomy. Signs include pyrexia (for which paracetamol may be given), flushing and sweating. There is usually a tachycardia, sometimes atrial fibrillation and high output cardiac failure. Propranolol, verapamil and digoxin may be used to treat the cardiac problems. Patients are often confused, restless or delirious and require sedation with a benzodiazepine or anti-psychotic medication such as chlorpromazine. In addition, the patients may require active cooling, rehydration with intravenous fluids, supplementary oxygen and antithyroid medication.

54 Porphyrias — Answers: B D E

The porphyrias are a group of inherited metabolic diseases in which there is an abnormality of porphyrin metabolism. Haem of haemoglobin contains a central porphyrin ring. If abnormally metabolised the porphyric patient may suffer an acute attack, which may be precipitated by a number of drugs including, classically, the barbiturates such as thiopentone or methohexitone, benzodiazepines and steroids. Propofol, opiates, muscle relaxants and all the volatile agents are thought to be safe. In addition bupivacaine and probably lignocaine are safe, and a regional technique is often advised.

55 Sensory signs — Answers: A B C E

Motor neurone disease, as the name implies, affects only motor neurones and there are no sensory signs.

In multiple sclerosis there are often sensory symptoms and signs. It may present with retro bulbar neuritis or paraesthesia and numbness in a limb.

Carpal tunnel syndrome is due to compression of the median nerve at the wrist as it passes deep to the flexor retinaculum. It produces pain and sensory signs in the distribution of the median nerve in the hand.

Tabes dorsalis is caused by tertiary syphilis and presents with signs of damage to the dorsal columns of the spinal cord, such as ataxia.

Syringomyelia is caused by an expanding cavity within the spinal cord which causes loss of pain and temperature sensation in the arms.

56 Phantom limb pain **Answers: A B**

Phantom limb pain is difficult to treat. It may be worsened by spinal anaesthesia. There is some weak evidence that the incidence may be reduced by establishing an epidural block some days prior to amputation. Systemic opioids are generally ineffective, but intrathecal opioids are sometimes successful.

57 A retrobulbar block **Answers: A C E**

In a retrobulbar block, local anaesthetic is injected within the muscle cone around the orbit, whereas in a peribulbar block the injection is outside the muscle cone. Within the muscle cone lie the optic, oculomotor, abducent and nasociliary (short and long ciliary) nerves. Thus all these nerves, except the optic nerve (which has a dural sheath), are blocked in a retrobulbar block.

With a retrobulbar block a separate facial nerve block is required and orbital akinesia is produced within 5 min.

A peribulbar block takes longer (15–30 min) and requires a greater volume of local anaesthetic, but may be associated with fewer serious complications, such as perforation of the globe. A separate facial nerve block is unnecessary.

Ref: Berry C B and Murphy P M. Regional anaesthesia for cataract surgery. *Br J Hosp Med* 1993; **49**(10): 689–701.

Ref: Johnson R W. Anatomy for ophthalmic anaesthesia. *Br J Anaesth* 1995; **75**: 80–87.

58 Sensory innervation of the hand **Answers: A B**

The sensation of the palm of the hand is supplied by the median and ulnar nerves. The median nerve supplies sensation to the thenar eminence and the palmar aspect of the radial three and a half digits, while the ulnar nerve supplies sensation to the rest of the palmar surface of the hand.

59 Coronary artery blood flow **Answers: A B C D**

Coronary artery blood flow occurs mainly in diastole. As heart rate increases the length of diastole decreases and thus tachycardia reduces coronary blood flow. If venous pressure rises the left ventricular end-diastolic pressure rises and myocardial wall tension increases leading to reduced coronary blood flow. Coronary artery blood flow is autoregulated and controlled by local mediators such as hydrogen ions, potassium ions and nitric oxide. Blood flow is increased by hypoxia.

60 The blood–brain barrier (BBB) **Answers: A B E**

The blood–brain barrier (BBB) forms a barrier between the cerebral circulation and the brain tissue. Lipid-soluble drugs such as fentanyl rapidly cross the BBB. Highly ionised drugs such as the quaternary amine neostigmine cannot cross. Tertiary amines, however, such as atropine and hyoscine, do cross the BBB. L-Dopa crosses the BBB where it is converted to dopamine which does not cross. Mannitol is given to treat cerebral oedema. As it does not normally cross the BBB it acts as an osmotic diuretic and draws water across the BBB and into the vascular space by osmosis.

61 Speed of uptake of an anaesthetic agent **Answer: B**

The speed of uptake of an anaesthetic agent is proportional to the minute ventilation and inversely proportional to the cardiac output and the blood gas solubility coefficient. It is unrelated to the MAC and is not temperature dependent.

62 Ketamine **Answers: C D E**

Ketamine is a phencyclidine derivative, presented as a racemic mixture.

It produces a unique state of dissociative anaesthesia. It is an antagonist at the NMDA receptor and also has actions at adrenergic, muscarinic, serotoninergic and opioid receptors. Its useful actions include potent analgesia, a sympathomimetic effect and a bronchodilator action. It is particularly indicated as an induction agent in the shocked or septic patient and the severe asthmatic. Side-effects include hypersalivation, increased intraocular and intracranial pressure and disturbing emergence reactions.

Ref: Hirota K and Lambert D G. Ketamine: its mechanism(s) of action and unusual clinical uses. *Br J Anaesth* 1996; **77**: 441–444.

63 Supraclavicular brachial plexus block — Answers: A B C D

Arterial puncture is another recognised complication.

64 Axillary brachial plexus block — Answer: A

There are three commonly used routes to block the brachial plexus: the axillary, interscalene and supraclavicular. The axillary route is probably the safest, while the supraclavicular is associated with a significant chance of pneumothorax. Other hazards of the supraclavicular route include subclavian artery puncture, and damage to the phrenic nerve, recurrent laryngeal and the cervical sympathetic trunk. The interscalene block is the most likely of the three routes to lead to either subarachnoid or extradural injection of local anaesthetic. The other main hazard with this route is injection into the vertebral artery.

65 Intercostal block — Answers: A B C

With an intercostal block the local anaesthetic is deposited between the internal and innermost intercostal muscles, in the subcostal groove, where the neurovascular bundle lies. Injected local anaesthetic will spread both to the opposite side and up and down one or two segments.

Bilateral blocks are contraindicated because of the risk of pneumothorax.

66 Caudal anaesthesia — Answers: B E

The caudal space is the sacral continuation of the extradural space. As the dural sac ends at S2 it is possible to enter the subarachnoid space with a caudal injection. The needle used for the caudal should not be inserted beyond a depth of 2–3 mm once the sacrococcygeal membrane has been pierced. Although far less likely, puncture of the fetal head has been reported. A catheter technique can be used in the caudal canal. The failure rate for caudals is higher than for other types of epidurals and because of the larger volume of the caudal space a greater volume of local anaesthetic is required to produce a given block than would be necessary for a lumbar epidural.

67 Epidural test dose — Answers: B E

An epidural test dose is used to detect inadvertent intravenous or subarachnoid injection. If a test dose is given intrathecally it produces a rapid, dense motor block in the legs. Intravenous injection may produce no effect, however. The patient sometimes complains of peri-oral paraesthesia or light headedness. If adrenaline is added to the test dose then intravenous injection may produce a tachycardia. However since there are many causes of tachycardia this is not a very specific test. An epidural test dose will delay rather than hasten the onset of analgesia. It in no way prevents neurological complications, nor does it prevent tachyphylaxis, which is simply a property of the local anaesthetic.

68 Pacemakers affected by anaesthetic drugs — Answers: A D E

Pacemakers may be affected by anaesthetic drugs, MRI scanners, shivering, diathermy and many other factors. Bipolar diathermy is safer than unipolar. MRI scanning is absolutely contraindicated in pacemaker patients. A magnet placed over a demand pacemaker will convert it to fixed-rate mode.

69 Moffet's solution — Answers: A B C

Moffet's solution contains 10% (100 mg/ml) cocaine. This is combined with adrenaline at a concentration of 0.1 mg/ml and 1% bicarbonate. The adrenaline intensifies the vasoconstrictor effect of the cocaine but increases the level of circulating catecholamines, predisposing to arrhythmias. In combination with halothane and hypercarbia in, for example, a spontaneously ventilating patient the result may be ventricular fibrillation. Moffet's is not used as analgesia. The safe maximum dose for cocaine when applied to the nasal mucosa is 1.5 mg/kg.

Ref: Nicholson K E and Rogers J E. Cocaine and adrenaline paste: a fatal combination? *Br Med J* 1995; **311**: 250–251.

70 Post-partum headache — Answers: A B C D E

Post-partum headache is most often non-pathological (cephalgia fugax).

Post dural puncture headache (PDPH) occurs in around 1% of mothers post spinal or epidural. The headache is typically aggravated by the upright posture and may be relieved by abdominal compression.

Treatment may involve an epidural blood patch. Although rare, headache may be caused by subarachnoid haemorrhage or cortical vein thrombosis. Herpes simplex encephalitis may cause headache, convulsions and pyrexia. The CSF reveals a lymphocytosis and CT or MRI scanning show abnormalities in the temporal lobes. Treatment is with intravenous acyclovir.

71 Bier's block **Answer: C**

Because of its cardiotoxicity bupivacaine is contraindicated for a Bier's block. Prilocaine is the agent of choice; it may cause methaemoglobinaemia, not carboxyhaemoglobinaemia. Although a double tourniquet technique is often used it is not mandatory. The cuff should be inflated to 100 mmHg above systolic pressure and should not be deflated until at least 20 min after injection of local anaesthetic.

72 Caudal epidural block **Answers: A B C D**

The complications of caudal block include motor weakness, infection, delayed micturition and nausea and vomiting. Accidental intravenous or intraosseous injection can lead to systemic toxicity while dural puncture produces a high or even total spinal block.

73 Complex regional pain syndrome type 1 **Answers: A B C D**

Complex regional pain syndrome type 1 (CRPS 1) was formerly known as reflex sympathetic dystrophy (RSD) or Sudeck's atrophy. CRPS II was formerly known as causalgia. CRPS type 1 involves sensory, motor and autonomic dysfunction. There may be osteoporosis and muscle atrophy in the affected limb. Allodynia (pain from normally innocuous stimuli), hyperalgesia (normally painful stimuli cause severe pain), skin pallor, sweating and goose flesh can all be seen. Therapeutic sympathetic blocks (stellate ganglion blocks, for example) and guanethidine blocks are used to treat CRPS type 1.

74 Maternal mortality **Answers: A C D E**

There were a total of 261 direct and indirect maternal deaths, representing an overall mortality rate of 13 in 100 000. Overall the commonest cause of death was suicide (classified as indirect). Of the direct deaths the commonest cause was thromboembolism, followed by hypertensive disorders, haemorrhage, and amniotic fluid embolism.

Anaesthesia was directly responsible for 6 deaths, an increase on the previous triennium, all associated with general anaesthesia.

Ref: *Report on Confidential Enquiries into Maternal Deaths in the United Kingdom, 2000-2002* http://www.cemach.org.uk/publications/WMD2000_2002_ExecSumm.pdf.

75 Intrathecal opioids — Answers: A B D

The four classic side-effects of intrathecal opioids such as fentanyl are pruritus, nausea and vomiting, urinary retention and respiratory depression. Shivering may also occur. Respiratory depression may be severe enough to require naloxone. Pruritus is often mild but can be treated with a small dose of propofol or naloxone.

Ref: Chaney M A. Side effects of intrathecal and epidural opioids. *Can J Anaesth* 1995; **42**: 891–903.

76 Nitrous oxide — Answer: B

The pressure in a nitrous oxide cylinder is temperature dependent. At 20°C it is 54 bar. Because nitrous oxide is present as a saturated vapour above a liquid the cylinder pressure only begins to fall once there is only vapour remaining. The critical temperature of nitrous oxide is 36.5°C; Entonox has a critical temperature of –8°C. The filling ratio of nitrous oxide is 0.67. Although nitrous oxide may cause megaloblastic changes in the bone marrow after prolonged exposure this is not due to vitamin B_{12} deficiency.

77 Minimum alveolar concentration (MAC) — Answers: A E

MAC is reduced in the presence of nitrous oxide, premedication agents, myxoedema, with increasing age and atmospheric pressure. MAC is not affected by pregnancy or sex.

78 One-lung anaesthesia — Answers: A B C D E

One-lung anaesthesia leads to a large shunt, since half the pulmonary blood flow is to unventilated lung.

The shunt equation is:

$$\frac{Q_S}{Q_T} = \frac{(C_CO_2 - C_aO_2)}{(C_CO_2 - C_{\bar{v}}O_2)} = \text{shunt fraction}$$

C_cO_2 = Pulmonary vein oxygen content

$C_{\bar{v}}O_2$ = Mixed venous oxygen content

C_aO_2 (the oxygen content of arterial blood) is determined by the haematocrit and the oxygen tension of blood, P_aO_2, since:

$C_aO_2 = Hb \times 1.34 + (P_aO_2 \times 0.003)$

Thus the shunt equation can be rewritten as:-

$$\frac{Q_S}{Q_T} = \frac{C_CO_2 - [Hb + P_aO_2]}{(C_CO_2 - C_{\bar{v}}O_2)}$$

Thus the P_aO_2 depends on the haematocrit, cardiac output, mixed venous oxygen content and the amount of blood flow to the unventilated lung, the shunt fraction. The P_aO_2 depends, of course, on the inspired oxygen tension.

79 Mapleson classification **Answers: A B C D E**

In 1954 Mapleson devised a classification for the breathing systems in use. They were labelled A–D; the Mapleson F breathing system was classified later. The A system is the Magill (or Lack coaxial version). It is the most efficient for spontaneous ventilation. The D system is the Bain, and is the most efficient for controlled ventilation. The E system is the Ayres T-piece and is the paediatric system used for patients of 20 kg or less. This system was modified by Jackson–Rees, who added an open-ended bag. This became the Mapleson F breathing system.

80 Steroid treatment regimens **Answers: B C D E**

The current recommendations for steroid treatment are summarised in the table below:

Ref: Nicholson G, Burrin J M and Hall G M. Peri-operative steroid supplementation, *Anaesthesia* 1998; **53**: 1091–1104.

Table reproduced by kind permission of Blackwell Science Ltd.

Patients currently taking steroids <10 mg/day	Assume normal HPA response	Additional steroid cover not required
Patients currently taking steroids >10 mg/day	Minor surgery	25 mg hydrocortisone at induction
	Moderate surgery	Usual preoperative steroids + 25 mg hydrocortisone at induction + 100 mg/day for 24 h
	Major surgery	Usual preoperative steroids + 25 mg hydrocortisone at induction + 100 mg/day for 72 h

High dose	Give usual immunosuppressive doses during immunosuppression peri-operative period
Patients stopped taking steroids <3 months	Treat as if on steroids
Patients stopped taking steroids >3 months	No peri-operative steroids necessary

81 Oxygen therapy — Answers: A B C D

While oxygen is clearly of benefit for all the other causes, retrolental fibroplasia is actually caused by oxygen.

82 Apgar score — Answers: A B D

Dr Virginia Apgar, an American anaesthetist, designed a simple scoring system to assess neonatal well-being. Scores of 0, 1 or 2 are given to each of the following five variables:

(a) heart rate
(b) respiratory effort
(c) muscle tone
(d) reflex movement
(e) colour

A score out of 10 is reached, having been measured at 1 and 5 min after delivery of the baby's head.

83 Mannitol — Answers: B C D E

Mannitol is an alcohol, not a sugar. It may be used to prevent the hepatorenal syndrome in jaundiced patients. It is found in dantrolene, the specific therapy for malignant hyperpyrexia. It may be used in patients with cerebral oedema. Because it is a hypertonic solution it draws cerebral oedema into the vascular compartment by osmosis. This may lead, however, to circulatory overload. Also, if the blood–brain barrier is damaged and permeable there may be a paradoxical worsening of neurological status after administration of mannitol.

84 Negative nitrogen balance **Answers: B C E**

A catabolic state, with associated muscle breakdown and a negative nitrogen balance exists post surgery. It is also found in patients receiving steroids and in starvation. In acute renal failure there is a failure to excrete the nitrogenous waste products of metabolism, and a positive nitrogen balance.

85 Intra-operative bronchospasm **Answers: A B D E**

Bronchospasm may be precipitated by pharmacological means.

Morphine can cause histamine release, which may then cause bronchospasm and wheeze. Pethidine has a lesser potential for histamine release, and may be preferred to morphine as a premed in an asthmatic. Atracurium and suxamethonium can also cause histamine release. Neostigmine blocks the action of acetylcholine esterase and therefore is a parasympathomimetic. It may thus cause bronchospasm. Isoflurane, like all the other volatile agents, relaxes bronchial smooth muscle. Light anaesthesia and stimulation of the trachea or carina by an endotracheal tube may lead to bronchospasm.

86 Pregnancy **Answers: A D E**

Enormous physiological changes occur in pregnancy. There is an increase in tidal volume and a reduction in FRC, while vital capacity is unchanged. Alveolar ventilation is increased, and the maternal P_aCO_2 is reduced. Airway resistance is usually unaffected by pregnancy. There is an increase in fibrinogen with reduced fibrinolysis and thus a hypercoagulable state.

There is an increase in heart rate and stroke volume and thus an elevated cardiac output. A reduction in systemic vascular resistance means that, overall, blood pressure is unchanged (in the absence of pregnancy-induced hypertension, which is common). The syndrome of supine hypotension from aorto-caval compression occurs in about 20% of pregnant women from 20 weeks onwards. The blood volume increases about 40% by term: though the increase in plasma volume is greater than the increase in red cell mass, leading to the physiological anaemia of pregnancy.

From the anaesthetic perspective the implications of anaesthetising a pregnant woman depend on the maturity of the fetus. In the first trimester the problems of teratogenicity from the anaesthetic drugs is the major concern. However, there is no evidence that any of the commonly employed anaesthetic agents are teratogens.

After 20 weeks there may be aorto-caval compression. There is an increased risk of aspiration and difficult intubation in the obstetric population. All mothers undergoing caesarean section receive antacid prophylaxis in the form of a histamine type 2 receptor antagonist and sodium citrate.

87 Predisposing factors for pre-eclampsia include — Answers: A B C D E

The factors can be classified as maternal and fetal. Fetal conditions predisposing to eclampsia include: multiple pregnancy; placental hydrops; and hydatidiform mole. Maternal factors include: primagravida; age less than 20 or greater than 35; family history; previous pre-eclampsia; existing microvascular diseases such as migraine, hypertension and diabetes.

88 Advantages of regional technique for TURP — Answers: A B

The advantages are: reduced blood loss; better assessment of cerebral function; bladder perforation more easily recognised (abdominal pain and rigidity); postoperative analgesia; reduced incidence of DVT.

The disadvantages are: loss of dignity; technical failure; unsuppressed cough; hypotension; hypoventilation; obturator reflex not blocked; post dural puncture headache.

Avoidance of teratogens is important for women in the first trimester of pregnancy.

89 Anaphylactic reactions associated with anaesthesia — Answers: B C E

The commonest presentation is cardiovascular collapse, with bronchospasm and skin changes only slightly less common. Factors which increase severity include asthma, beta-blockade and neuraxial anaesthesia – all of these states are associated with a reduced endogenous catecholamine response. Elevated serum tryptase indicates that the reaction was associated with mast cell degranulation, and this occurs after both anaphylactic and anaphylactoid reactions.

Ref: *Suspected anaphylactic reactions associated with anaesthesia.* Association of Anaesthetists, 2003.

90 Oral hypoglycaemics **Answers: A E**

The sulfonylureas increase insulin secretion and include (shortest acting first) tolbutamide, glibenclamide, chlorpropamide and gliclazide. The highest risk of hypoglycaemia is with glibenclamide.

Metformin, a biguanide, increases insulin sensitivity and decreases hepatic gluconeogenesis. Hypoglycaemia is not a risk.

Acarbose, an α-glucosidase inhibitor, reduces the breakdown of starch to sugar in the gut.

Practice Paper 4: Clinical Viva Answers

Viva 1

Examiner 1

Please summarise this case
This is a 60-year-old ex-miner who has presented for open resection of a sigmoid carcinoma. He has severe restrictive and obstructive lung disease, and his breathing has worsened over the last few weeks, possibly related to a change in his medication, to a point where he is acutely unwell. From his history and examination there is a suggestion that there is also an element of untreated cardiac failure.

What information would you particularly like to find out by taking a history from this patient?
We need to find out what his level of fitness was before the recent deterioration.

The recent deterioration may be due to a respiratory or cardiac problem.

Respiratory causes may be due to a worsening of his COPD, and this may follow the temporal relationship of the reduction in his steroid dose. He may have a chest infection, and so should be asked about cough, sputum and fever.

How can you decide whether shortness of breath is due to a respiratory or cardiac cause?
The decision is based on a directed history, examination and set of investigations, but even then it can be very difficult to tease out the major factor in some cases.

In the history orthopnoea, paroxysmal nocturnal dyspnoea (PND) and ankle swelling point towards a cardiac cause; relief with bronchodilators suggests COPD; and fever and productive cough, infection. Exertional dyspnoea, wheeze and general cough are reasonably non-specific.

On examination hyperinflation and prolonged expiratory phase suggest a COPD, localised crepitations and fever suggest infection and oedema suggests cardiac. The presence of fine basal crepitations may signify wet, oedematous lungs, or may be due to pulmonary fibrosis.

Key investigations include peak expiratory flow rate, formal lung function tests, chest X-ray, ECG and cardiac echocardiography. On chest X-ray you might specifically expect to see an enlarged heart, the alveolar shadowing of pulmonary oedema, fluid in the fissures and pleural effusions in heart failure. A low ejection fraction on cardiac echo may help to rule in a cardiac cause, but may not rule out a respiratory component.

Describe the chest X-ray to me
This is a PA chest X-ray of --- taken on ---. The most obvious features are of widespread reticular lung field shadowing, consistent with a diagnosis of pulmonary fibrosis. There is no evidence of heart failure, in that there is no evidence of upper lobe diversion, fluid in the fissures, pleural effusion or Kerley B lines and the heart is of normal size.

Describe the ECG to me
This is a normal ECG. The rate is 70 beats/min; it is sinus rhythm; there is no QRS axis deviation and no evidence of old or current ischaemia.

What do you make of the arterial blood gas? What were you expecting the arterial blood gas to be? How can you explain this arterial blood gas?
This is an entirely normal blood gas. It is surprising given the clinical picture and the severity of disease shown in the lung function tests and X-ray. It might be expected that the pO_2 would be lower (7–8 kPa), and the pCO_2 and HCO_3 higher.

One explanation is that this gas has been mislabelled, and is not from the expected patient [this is probably an important observation, which shows understanding of the real world]. The pO_2 may be higher than expected if the patient was receiving supplemental oxygen (although it has been labelled 'on air'). The 'normal' pCO_2 probably does not reflect an acute reduction from a higher level as the HCO_3 is not raised and the pH is normal.

Are you ready to anaesthetise him today?
No. This man is acutely unwell, with a high risk of peri-operative mortality. He should be admitted to hospital for review and further investigations of his chest and heart under the general physicians. Stabilisation of this acute condition and a return to his previous 'best' level of functioning will reduce his peri-operative risk.

I will speak to the surgeon and the patient and discuss my findings and plans. I understand that as this is an urgent operation for tumour resection the surgical team will want to operate as soon as is possible, and it would be useful to have an indication as to how long they are prepared to wait.

He is now optimised, describe your anaesthetic
The major issues here are:

- Surgical – laparotomy requiring muscle relaxation, a large incision requiring good analgesia, bowel prep causing dehydration, and an operating time of 2+ hours making fluid balance and heat loss problems
- Patient – severe respiratory disease, with an FEV_1 of 0.7 l making ventilation and weaning difficult; probable underlying cardiac disease; a bowel tumour making malnourishment likely; sub-acute obstruction and delayed gastric emptying time a potential problem.

The anaesthetic aim is that by the end of the operation he is warm, pain free, well filled and haemodynamically stable, enabling the option of early extubation.

Having placed a large peripheral intravenous line and a thoracic epidural at T9 I would place an arterial line to monitor BP and enable ABG evaluation of peri-operative ventilation and acid–base status. If I thought he did not need a rapid sequence induction I would induce him with midazolam, fentanyl, propofol and atracurium, maintaining the starting blood pressure with vasopressors. Maintenance of anaesthesia will be with a mixture of oxygen, air and sevoflurane, together with the analgesia provided by the epidural. Having intubated him I would pass an NG tube and temperature probe. I would insert an internal jugular central line. I would use an oesophageal Doppler to help guide fluid replacement. In theatre I would set up a fluid warmer and warming blanket.

At the end of the operation, if surgery had been straightforward and the anaesthetic aims met, I would extubate him sitting up and transfer to the high-dependency unit for postoperative recovery.

Would you aim to ventilate him postoperatively?
Ideally he should be ventilated for as short a time as possible to try to avoid ventilator-associated pneumonia and atrophy of the muscles of respiration. The fear with this patient is that having started mechanical ventilation he will be impossible to wean from it.

Clinical short cases

Examiner 2

1. *You are on-call one Saturday night at your labour ward. There is a commotion in the corridor and a midwife runs up to you and says that an unbooked woman has just been brought in bleeding per vagina.*

What is the differential diagnosis?
- <28 weeks – abortion, lower genital tract causes (cervical polyps, erosions, etc)
- >28 weeks 'antepartum haemorrhage' – placental abruption/praevia; 'post-partum' – uterine atony (including retained products), uterine rupture, trauma.

What do you do first?
This is an emergency, obstetric haemorrhage is potentially fatal.

ABC – check the airway is clear, put on 100% O_2, check ventilation, put on S_pO_2 probe, assess pulse, BP and capillary refill, place two large-bore IV lines taking blood for FBC and cross-match. Call the obstetrician urgently.

The obstetric registrar says she thinks that the woman has placental abruption and needs an emergency caesarean section.

Describe your anaesthetic.
The options for caesarean are regional or general anaesthesia. General anaesthesia is faster and enables easier control of blood pressure, and therefore my choice in this situation assuming no contraindications. The bleeding may be very heavy requiring warm fluid infusers and invasive monitoring.

I will call for extra help, then take a short history of allergies and medical and anaesthetic problems, and assess the airway. I would give sodium citrate. Having made sure the IV lines were working well, preparations were being made for major transfusion, and the surgeons were scrubbed and ready, I would prepare for a rapid sequence induction in theatre when she was cleaned and draped in left lateral tilt.

What induction agent would you use for general anaesthesia?
I would induce with thiopentone and suxamethonium. Etomidate could be an alternative, causing slightly less hypotension, but as the thiopentone is already drawn up and I am used to using it, it would be my choice.

How would you maintain anaesthesia?
I would maintain anaesthesia with isoflurane 1% in oxygen and atracurium. After delivery of the fetus I would give incremental doses of fentanyl to provide analgesia and consider increasing the isoflurane as her blood pressure will tolerate to 1.3 MAC.

2. *You have just delivered a fit and well 35-year-old woman to the recovery ward extubated following a straightforward hysterectomy.*

You are just relaxing in the coffee room when a recovery nurse comes in and says the woman you have just left appears to be very confused.

What would you do?
Go and see her.
ABC.
Then determine the cause with history, examination and investigations, and correct it.

What is the differential diagnosis?
A 'surgical sieve' type answer is best here

Physiological – hypoxia, hypercarbia, hypotension (all causes of shock), hypo/hyperthermia

Pharmacological – opiates, benzos, residual anaesthetic agents (or withdrawal, eg alcohol)

Biochemical – hypoglycaemia, acidaemia, electrolyte imbalance, high urea/bilirubin

In the head things – CVA, epilepsy, tumour, trauma (subdural)

The recovery staff do an ECG (Fig. 12)
Fig. 12 shows a narrow complex regular tachycardia (supra ventricular tachycardia) with a rate of 180 beats/min.

What is your management?
By the 2005 Resuscitation Council guidelines her reduced consciousness puts her into the 'unstable' group, the treatment of which is synchronised DC shock under sedation followed by amiodarone 300 mg IV over 10–20 min.

If there is time it may be possible to try vagal manoeuvres or adenosine first.

3. *That afternoon you are anaesthetising for a urology list. The first patient is an 80-year-old man for transurethral resection of a bladder tumour. The surgeon sees you just before you go off to pre-assess the first patient and says that he is worried about the patient moving due to obturator nerve stimulation if you do a regional technique.*

What are the anaesthetic options?
Paralysis with a neuromuscular blocking agent is the only choice to stop movement on stimulating the obturator nerve (although theoretically a local anaesthetic block of the nerve distal to the stimulation may also work). The anaesthetic options are to paralyse and ventilate with either an LMA or an endotracheal tube, with or without a regional block to provide analgesia.

Your patient's blood pressure is 180/120 mmHg today

Would you anaesthetise him today?
A diastolic of >120 mmHg (on repeated readings over a period of time) is classified as severe hypertension.

The first thing is to go and recheck his blood pressure myself, and compare it to any previously recorded readings, eg from pre-assessment clinic or previous admissions.

There are three problems. Firstly the cause of the hypertension is unknown, it is probably essential, but there could be another cause such as renal failure. Secondly there may be end-organ damage, eg heart, kidney, brain, eyes. Lastly the blood pressure is likely to be more labile during anaesthesia, and there will be an increased rate of associated morbidity and mortality (MI, CVA, renal failure).

Although peri-operative risks are increased with lesser levels of hypertension it has been found that in the absence of end-organ damage then these risks are not reduced even after the hypertension is treated.

But in this case, if the blood pressure is severely high on repeated measurement, and with agreement from the surgical team, then today's procedure should be postponed for diagnosis and treatment of this hypertension.

How long would you delay the surgery for?
The pressure should ideally be controlled for several weeks before the operation.

Viva 2 (Clinical Sciences)

Examiner 1

What is a transducer?

How does an invasive blood pressure transducer work?

Draw a Wheatstone bridge

What are resonance and damping?

What is critical damping and signal-to-noise ratio?

Transducers – devices that convert one form of energy to another.

Arterial transducers have a piezoelectric strain gauge applied to the surface of a flexible diaphragm which bulges in response to transmitted changes in arterial pressure. When the piezoelectric quartz crystal is deformed a voltage is generated across its faces as a result. This small amplitude signal is amplified using a bridge circuit.

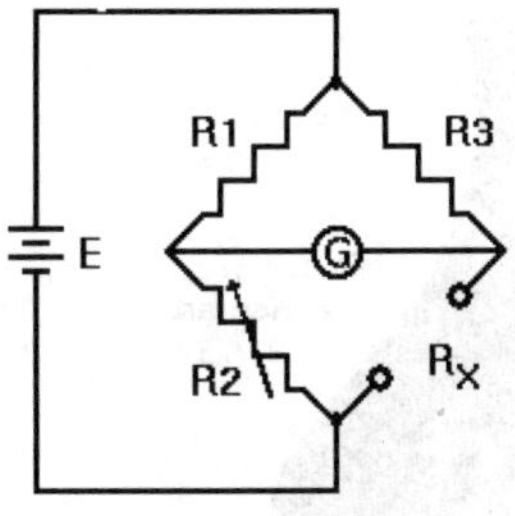

A Wheatstone bridge

Resonance – the situation where an oscillating system responds with maximal amplitude to an external driving force.

Damping – a reduction in the amplitude of oscillations in a resonant system.

Critical damping – in measurement systems this is the level of damping which gives the fastest response, without overshoot, to a change in the measured quantity.

Signal-to-noise ratio – the log of the amplitude of the 'noise' divided by the amplitude of the signal – measured in dB.

What is the sensory innervation of the head?

What are the branches of the ophthalmic division of the trigeminal nerve?

How might you block them?

What other nerve blocks of the face do you know?

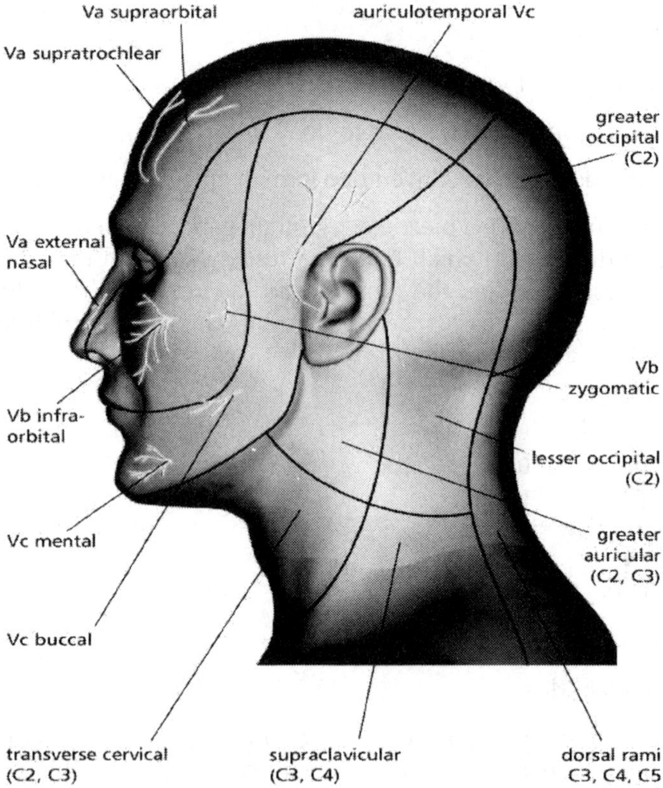

Sensation to the face and forehead are supplied by the trigeminal (V) nerve. All three divisions can be blocked by a block of the Gasserian (trigeminal)

ganglion, which can be accessed by passing a needle through the foramen ovale with X-ray guidance.

The three major branches of the ophthalmic division pass through the superior orbital fissure:

- The lacrimal nerve supplies the lateral upper eyelid and conjunctiva
- The frontal nerve has two branches:
  - supraorbital – frontal sinuses, anterior scalp and part of the upper eyelid
  - supratrochlear – medial forehead and upper eyelid
- The nasociliary nerve
  - anterior ethmoidal – external skin of nose, upper anterior nasal cavity, anterior ethmoids
  - posterior ethmoidal – posterior ethmoidal, sphenoid sinuses
  - infratrochlear – medial upper eyelid and conjunctiva
  - long ciliary nerves – to ciliary ganglion

Blocks

- supraorbital: 2 ml 2% lignocaine injected at the supraorbital notch
- supratrochlear: 2 ml at the superiomedial part of the orbit
- (4 ml subcutaneous infiltration above the eyebrow will also block both of the above)
- frontal: 1 ml in the central part of the roof of the orbit.

Examiner 2

Tell me about the effects of hypothermia

- Metabolic: reduced BMR so reduced CO_2 production and O_2 consumption, reduced drug metabolism, hyperglycaemia common
- Respiratory: shivering increases oxygen consumption fivefold, left shift of oxyhaemoglobin dissociation curve, decreased pulmonary hypoxic vasoconstriction, reduction in respiratory rate
- Cardiovascular: myocardial depression, bradycardia, hypotension, J waves on ECG, risk of VF below 28°C
- CNS: reduction in consciousness below 30°C, reduction in cerebral blood flow (but also of cerebral oxygen demand)
- Renal: reduced GFR but urine output usually maintained by reduced ADH and tubular reabsorption
- Anaesthetic: reduction of MAC, vasoconstriction causes problems with pulse oximetry

Please classify antidepressant drugs

For each class explain how they work, their side-effects, what problems they cause in overdose, and if they have special implications for anaesthetists

Class	**Example**	**Action**	**Side-effects**	**Overdose**	**Anaesthesia**
Tricyclics	Clomipramine Amitriptyline	Prevent NA, dopamine (and 5-HT) reuptake at synapse (also antagonise mACh, H_1, α_1)	Sedation Anticholinergic effects Arrhythmias	CV: tachycardia, hypotension, ^PR, ^QT to give AF, VT, VF, heart block Other: agitation, hyper-reflexia, convulsions, coma	Increased sensitivity to catecholamines, increased risk of arrhythmias
MAOI	Iproniazid Phenelzine Pargyline Moclobemide	Antagonise the breakdown of monoamine neurotransmitters after uptake into nerve terminals	Inability to break down exogenous amines Cheese reaction (sertraline tyramine)		? stop for 3 weeks Unpredictable response to vasoconstrictors (especially indirect) Pethidine may cause coma
SSRI	Fluoxetine Paroxetine Sertraline	Prevent 5-HT reuptake at synapse	Diarrhoea, nausea, headache, anxiety	Serotonin syndrome may occur if taken with tricyclics or MAOIs	Pethidine may provoke serotonin syndrome
Lithium	Lithium Therapeutic range 0.4–1.0 mmol/l	Displaces intracellular K^+, cells less depolarised, easier to reach threshold potential	Inhibits ADH, polyuria Hypothyroid Thirst, tremor, weakness Arrhythmias	Tremor, ataxia, GIT upset, weakness, twitching Hypokalaemia, arrhythmias, renal failure, convulsions, coma	Stop 3 days before Potentiates non-depolarising muscle relaxants Delays the action of suxamethonium

INDEX

This book has been indexed by question. Each locator consists of the question type, paper number and question number. For example, SA2.11 is short answer question number 11 in paper 2, MC3.36 is multiple choice question number 36 in paper 3 and V4.1 is viva number 1 in paper 4.